MY THREE YEAR JOURNEY
— TO THE —
NEW YORK CITY MARATHON

AN INSPIRATIONAL JOURNAL
(JOURNEY)

HAE S. BOLDUC

BALBOA.PRESS
A DIVISION OF HAY HOUSE

Copyright © 2022 Hae S. Bolduc.

All rights reserved. No part of this book may be used or reproduced by any means, graphic, electronic, or mechanical, including photocopying, recording, taping or by any information storage retrieval system without the written permission of the author except in the case of brief quotations embodied in critical articles and reviews.

Balboa Press books may be ordered through booksellers or by contacting:

Balboa Press
A Division of Hay House
1663 Liberty Drive
Bloomington, IN 47403
www.balboapress.com
844-682-1282

Because of the dynamic nature of the Internet, any web addresses or links contained in this book may have changed since publication and may no longer be valid. The views expressed in this work are solely those of the author and do not necessarily reflect the views of the publisher, and the publisher hereby disclaims any responsibility for them.

The author of this book does not dispense medical advice or prescribe the use of any technique as a form of treatment for physical, emotional, or medical problems without the advice of a physician, either directly or indirectly. The intent of the author is only to offer information of a general nature to help you in your quest for emotional and spiritual well-being. In the event you use any of the information in this book for yourself, which is your constitutional right, the author and the publisher assume no responsibility for your actions.

Any people depicted in stock imagery provided by Getty Images are models, and such images are being used for illustrative purposes only. Certain stock imagery © Getty Images.

Print information available on the last page.

ISBN: 979-8-7652-3380-1 (sc)
ISBN: 979-8-7652-3379-5 (hc)
ISBN: 979-8-7652-3381-8 (e)

Library of Congress Control Number: 2022916045

Balboa Press rev. date: 10/20/2022

Contents - Journal Highlights

2019
Feb	New York City Marathon Acceptance	1
Apr	Boston Marathon	48
Jun	10-Mile Garden of the Gods Race	87
Aug	Pikes Peak Ascent	117
Oct	Beginning to Taper	148
Nov	New York City Marathon	163

2020
Mar	Detour	168
Jul	Nature's Way	174
Sep	High Colorado Mountains	182
Nov	New Birth	188

2021
Mar	New Year New Goal	190
Oct	Chicago Marathon	193
Nov	New York City Marathon	194

2022
Epilogue	200

Countdown 2019

Thursday, January 31, 2019
Colorado Springs, CO

I return home from an early-morning test run. The run went well, but I still felt a little soreness in my hip and decided to stop at 1.7 miles and attend to my business. I am a Lifestyle Coach, and the session with my client goes well. After the session, I sit down to take care of some personal business and read my email. I'm stunned and excited to see an email from the New York City Marathon officials. I qualified in 2018 and applied to participate. And here it is, my answer. I open the email to find that I have been accepted! I can't believe it. I love New York and everything about New York City. Every time I visit, I love the people, the culture, the food, and Grand Central Terminal. Participating in the marathon will allow me to discover the city in a different way and with a new perspective. I've heard stories for years of how difficult it is to get into the New York City Marathon. Only 50,000 out of more than 100,000 applicants are accepted each year. I feel elated to have this opportunity and also glad I've been giving my body a chance to rest and heal. Now my training will begin.

Countdown: 275 Days

Friday, February 1, 2019
Colorado Springs, CO

It's a beautiful day, sunny, and in the 50s. All the snow has melted and the trail is clear with no ice. Craig and I have returned from a trip to Arizona - Phoenix (in the 70s), Sedona (50s), Flagstaff (20s), and the South Rim of the Grand Canyon (20s). We often take short trips to explore areas we haven't experienced and we took this one to escape to a warmer clime for my Boston Marathon training. To be honest, I'm hurting after my 8-mile Colorado Springs Winter Series II Race this past Saturday. My right hip is giving me trouble and I'm surprised because this has never before happened. I'm a mindful runner and I always listen to my body. I was hoping this short getaway would allow me to heal. After the Winter Series II race and during our three-day visit to Arizona, I didn't run a single mile until the last day, giving my body total rest for four days.

Countdown: 274 Days
Saturday, February 2, 2019
Colorado Springs, CO

It's 8:30 a.m. and already 38°F and sunny. It's another beautiful day for running in Colorado Springs and I'm anxious to go out for a test run with my healing right hip. Everything takes time when it comes to healing one's body. All the cells are working 24-hours a day on their repair assignment, and I am so grateful. My mind is focused on my hip when I start running and I start slowly, tiptoeing to see how it will react. I feel tightness in my hip, but no pain. I run to the trail a block from our home and continue running to the corner of Centennial Blvd and Vindicator where the Ute Valley Park sign is located. This is exactly one mile in and I'm at 11 minutes and 30 seconds. Pretty darn slow. But I wasn't going for speed this morning. I intend to slow down and allow my body to recover. I continue running to Eagleview Middle School, about two miles from home before I turn back, still cautious about my hip. I run into Craig on the trail. He is just starting as I'm finishing. We used to run together, which was so much fun, but these days we have different purposes for our runs. Craig doesn't have any races scheduled this year, so most of the time he is on "exploratory" runs and he can't wait to tell me all about the new trails he discovers. He has been living in Colorado Springs for over 30 years and is now finally observing his surroundings and experiencing life at a deeper level. Before this, like everyone else, Craig and I were entrenched in our careers and families, buried under life happenings. We hardly had time to experience real life. I finish up at 4.8 miles and I am feeling good with no discomfort in any body parts. A good test-run day.

Countdown: 273 Days
Sunday, February 3, 2019
Colorado Springs, CO

My training for the Boston Marathon has not been smooth. Yes, I have been accepted into the Boston Marathon, on April 15, 2019, as well as the New York City Marathon, on November 3, 2019. I'm in for two big ones this year. There's a lot of excitement and pressure that comes with these two "major" marathons. I'm far from being an elite competitive runner; nevertheless, the nature of my character is to give 100% in everything I do. Therefore, it's my goal to train the best I can by following the plan my coach and husband, Craig, put together for me. I was very healthy until December 2018 and had never been hurt or injured from running or any other sport, for that matter. Well, that's not quite true. I'm a clumsy bike rider and tend to fall sometimes, bruising or scraping my knees and/or legs.

After the fourth and final Fall Series race last year—a local race series consisting of one race every other week starting in October—I felt some minor discomfort in my left iliotibial band (ITB). On race day, November 11th, we woke up to eight inches of wet, sloppy snow. The racecourse was icy, muddy, and slippery. I fell five times but had a soft landing each time. I didn't feel any discomfort in my body at any time during the day. About a week later, I started feeling my left ITB tighten up and a sharp jolt of pain down my left leg. I had never been in this situation, though I had heard or read countless stories in running magazines and books about running injuries.

The ITB injury caused sharp shooting pain down my leg when I ran, so in December I slowed down my running both in distance and speed. December went by and I was feeling good at the beginning of the year. I jumped into my Boston Marathon training, which included the Winter Series, a four-race series with a race every other week starting in January. Each race was progressively longer: 10 km, 8 miles, 10 miles, and 20 km. I ran two hard training runs, a 10-mile run, and a 12-mile run before Saturday's 8-mile race. Although I took a rest on Friday, it was not enough. After Saturday's race, my right hip was hurting.

Today, I was planning on running a local half-marathon as my long training run but instead, I'm "sitting" out the day. As much as I adhere to the book "Love What Is" by Byron Katie, this sidelined feeling is hard to swallow. Instead of feeling bad about not running the half-marathon today, I'll focus on Boston, starting tomorrow. My body is sending me a clear message to focus on "quality" rather than "quantity" so I will listen to my body and heal. Our bodies are amazing machines and in every moment miracles are taking place. For that I am grateful.

Countdown: 272 Days

Monday, February 4, 2019

<u>Colorado Springs, CO</u>

It is early February, and the temperature is in the 40s which makes for beautiful running weather in the morning sun. On the trail, I can see the trees yawning and beginning to wake up from their winter nap. I hear and see signs of spring; birds are chirping and squirrels are leading me into Ute Valley Park, a wooded 500-acre undeveloped parkland. Several shady areas in the park still have thick ice and I end up running around one of these locations, just off the edge of the trail, to avoid slipping. It is so fun to run this morning, albeit slowly, after a week of downtime. The southwest corner of the Ute Valley Park trail merges into the flat neighborhood Piñon Valley Park, where I'll see if I can do some actual running. The sidewalk loop around the park is one-third of a mile. I run hard for three loops and find it fun and pain-free. Running without pain or discomfort feels like freedom and leaves me feeling thankful.

I am continuously learning how to treat the one body I have with respect and nourishing food. Craig and I have been on a whole food plant-based lifestyle since 2014, after discovering the "The China Study," a book by T. Collin Campbell. We avoid meat, eggs, dairy, and processed foods including all oils, refined sugar, and salt. Craig's "famous" 21-ingredient, oatmeal-blueberry pancakes with organic berry, raisin, and walnut compote have nourished my body before the morning training run today and, afterward, I make a green smoothie with kale, spinach, chard, avocado, celery, ginger, turmeric, banana, and black pepper. Lunch and dinner are packed with whole grains, lentils, quinoa, a variety of beans, sweet potatoes, and an assortment of veggies to satisfy Dr. Joel Fuhrman's G-BOMBS, which stands for greens, beans, onions, mushrooms, berries, and seeds plus grains. We also love Michael Greger's "How Not to Die Cookbook." We both love sweets consisting of dried fruits, fresh fruits, and homemade desserts, such as No-Bake Brownies from Greger's cookbook made with cacao, walnuts, and dates. We add flaxseeds, pumpkin seeds, sunflower seeds, and goji berries to various dishes.

It has been our journey to live healthy in mind, body, and spirit. We love to share the nutritional information we have learned with those who are interested, and it's rewarding to see people make changes and watch their health improve. Our Holistic Health Retreat Airbnb has been a perfect venue to introduce receptive guests to plant-based whole foods. Even if we can make a small impact on our friends, family, community, or even strangers, our life is enhanced.

Countdown: 271 Days

Tuesday, February 5, 2019

Colorado Springs, CO

My Boston Marathon training schedule was developed by my coach, my best friend, my husband, and my lover. It is a 4:3:2 schedule with four days of running, three days of strength training, and two days of yoga per week. I love my yoga sessions on Tuesday and Thursday evenings. My yoga instructor is a true gift. She is so gentle with just the right amount of encouragement to push me. It is the goldilocks approach, not too much and not too little. If a movement hurts anywhere, she asks us to back off. How cool is that? Pain is no fun. Our class size usually runs between six and

20 people and is conducted with gentle yoga music in a warm candlelight setting. It's truly a time to relax, scan the body, and breathe deeply to release stress and tension. We live in this busy, on-the-go society. It's not easy to take time to "let go of the day" and get ready for the night's rest so we can wake up fresh in the morning. The yoga studio is only two miles from home, and sometimes I jog or run over for the yoga session if Craig happens to be using the car.

Craig and I are minimalists, which doesn't mean getting rid of every material thing you own. What minimalism means to us is owning only those things that make us happy. Craig and I are both in our second marriage and, when we merged, we had many duplicate cooking pots, kitchen utensils, books, bedding items, towels, etc. We sold the valuable items and donated many others. During this process, we also sold my car. We only have one car now, but own three bicycles: one mountain bike each, and a tandem bike we call Cappuccino after the coffee we once enjoyed so much. When we are out on Cappuccino, we use our coffee commands as follows: black for "stop," espresso for "go," and latte for "slow down." Lately, we've been focusing so much on running that poor Cappuccino is covered with dust and the tires are flat after sitting so long without use. She's in the garage, patiently waiting for her turn to go out on the road again when we slow down our running training. I wonder when that might be?

Countdown: 270 Days

Wednesday, February 6, 2019

<u>Colorado Springs, CO</u>

It's late for me this morning. My Wednesday Toastmasters meeting is over at 8:00. I delivered a speech on mentor/mentee relationships and was delighted to win the best speaker award. Toastmasters International, a nonprofit international organization, has become a life force for me since I first joined in 2008. I began my Toastmasters journey to improve my public speaking and leadership skills. I was petrified when I gave my first speech. I was sick to my stomach and had to call in sick to work. Since then, I have grown and enjoy speaking in front of an audience.

I get home from the meeting and change into running clothes to do a speed workout. We have a half-mile straight, slightly downhill, gravel trail near our home and I can do fast half-mile intervals with slow half-mile jogs in between. Today, I was able to do five half-mile intervals. The sun was out and the wind was blowing into my face. Thankfully, I'd worn my windbreaker and didn't feel cold.

I "ran" into our recently retired neighbor walking his chocolate Labradoodle. He's a wonderful guy. Every time it snows even a small amount, he comes over with his snow blower and cleans our driveway. We live in a neighborhood with outstanding neighbors, including Randy and Linda "North" and Randy and Linda "South." Yup, two couples have the same names on each side of our home. Randy and Linda North have a beautiful garden in the summer and share their garden veggies with us, including chard, radish, and squash. They are omnivores but know Craig and I consume huge quantities of veggies.

Countdown: 269 Days

Thursday, February 7, 2019

<u>Colorado Springs, CO</u>

    I had grocery shopping duty today since Craig needed time to work on our taxes. Divide and conquer is our motto. I have been so lucky that Craig has been doing the food shopping all these years. I didn't realize how exhausting it is. To me, buying groceries is a waste of time and hard-earned money. But we do love to eat, so someone has to do the dirty work. I am completely drained after shopping and running three miles at an 8-minute/mile pace on the treadmill at the gym this morning. It was only 2°F outside, and with the slippery, snow-covered streets I decided to run indoors. I love treadmill running. Many people find it mentally grueling, but I love the controlled temperature. Plus, there's no wind resistance and no rocks or other obstacles. I just plug into some good music and have at it. After my run, I stretched and sat in the hot sauna. It felt great, especially on this cold winter morning.

    I used to dislike the idea of paying for a gym membership. My thinking was, why pay to work out when I'm the one doing all the work? But moving to Colorado Springs where winter days can be harsh with snow, wind, and cold weather changed my mind. And, luckily, there was a gym only two miles from our home. I joined, and I have no regrets. Now, I have my choice of running on the trails, roads, or treadmill, and doing strength training, too. Plus, there's that sauna. Life is so gratifying.

Countdown: 268 Days

Friday, February 8, 2019

<u>Colorado Springs, CO</u>

Today, I'm giving my body a 100% rest. It's been a while since I took a total break. I'm not even going to stretch. Just let it be. I'm grateful for the opportunity of a much-deserved break, as tomorrow I'll run the 10-mile Winter Series III race.

Normally, I'd be following my routine race ritual today. The day before a race, I usually feel calm. I scan my body to see how it feels then I either do strength training or a three to 4-mile shakeout run. On the morning of the race, I get up and have one piece of toasted Ezekiel bread with peanut butter, honey, and banana. I drink one 8-ounce cup of coffee. Then I do gratitude journaling as I'm always very thankful to have the ability to run and know that not everyone who wants to run can run. I depend on being strong to run safely and I accept everything as is—the weather, the trail conditions, and anything else I don't have control over. Local races are low-key to run and I get to meet and have fun running with other runners.

Countdown: 267 Days

Saturday, February 9, 2019

<u>Colorado Springs, CO</u>

The 10-mile Winter Series III race at Goose Gossage Park is less than five miles from our home. The weather is ideal for the race—36°F sunny, light wind, and a perfect venue. It is close to home with plenty of parking for the runners' and spectators' cars. The course is on an asphalt trail and feels fast to me after running gravel and rocky trails. There's always the option to run on the dirt trail along the edge of the asphalt, but all the runners I see are running on the pavement.

I woke up fresh after a good night's sleep and had my pre-race breakfast. At the bib pickup table, I see some familiar faces—Kevin and Rudy who are Craig's former age group competitors, and our best friends, Verena and John, who are running the short series 5-mile course today. I see Jennifer and Michelle, our Sunrise Strider running group friends, both smiling. Everyone is hyped up, happy, and ready for the race director's announcement. Ready, set, go. We're off, right at 10:00.

I find myself running behind three chatty ladies. They're running at a good tempo and I tune out their conversations, looking only at their footsteps. It is as if they are pacing me, and it's awesome to have not one, but three pacers. After eight miles, I have trouble keeping up with my pacers and fall behind. I see Phil passing me. What I need is a little more energy to push through the last two miles, but somehow, I am falling behind and more runners are passing me. I finish the 10-mile race at a 9:07 minute/mile pace. I feel I should have been able to push harder the last two miles, but I'm happy with my result. It's my longest run in weeks without hip pain; that alone is enough cause for me to celebrate. How fortunate I am to be able to run, and once again, I'm grateful for my strong, healthy body. Craig prepared a post-race lunch of beans, sweet potatoes, and greens. He's the best coach I've ever had. He takes care of all the logistics of getting to the races and the recovery food and rest. My personal one-stop-shopping coach.

Countdown: 266 Days

Sunday, February 10, 2019

<u>Colorado Springs, CO</u>

I love Sundays. Sundays are our "date day," the day Craig and I are committed to spending time together doing WHATEVER we like. Sometimes we explore a new place, sometimes we go out to a movie or concert, and sometimes we stay in and watch a good movie on Amazon Prime with all the comforts of home. We have an amazing relationship, and we adore each other. We respect each other's space and are playful when we are together. It's all good clean fun, as Craig puts it.

We also love to read books and share our thoughts on every chapter along the way. When we were plugged into the professional world, we always read books related to our profession. Now I enjoy reading books on running. I have already finished six running books this year and have several spiritual online library books queued up. I take advantage of the "Libby" iPhone app, digitally checking out and returning books from the Pikes Peak Library District.

Craig and I love to spend time together. Time may be limited for all of us, but one thing is for sure, our life and destiny are shaped by the person with whom we spend time. I have time this morning to strength train and stretch to aid my recovery from yesterday's race, and this afternoon we are heading out to a movie for our date day.

Countdown: 265 Days

Monday, February 11, 2019

<u>Colorado Springs, CO</u>

I have been drawn into Michael Singer's book, "The Surrender Experiment" and it's difficult to put down. The life lesson I've learned from the book is that the universe is clearly in charge. I'm learning to surrender to life's happenings instead of resisting the unknown or choosing my preferences over the flow of life. I must incorporate this life lesson into my daily activities—running, strength training, and all life challenges. I must simply observe the events unfolding, quietly think about what I am learning, and allow myself to go to new places.

Since reading the book, I have been asking myself the following questions, "What am I doing?" and "Why am I here?" I find these to be unbounded questions with no clear answers. I know one thing for sure, that I must devote more time to meditating to help clear my path in life. Surrender is not about moving in whatever direction the wind is blowing. I can't change the wind, but I can change the sail. Destiny is a universal force. However, I can change how I experience and learn from unfolding events by surrendering unconditionally.

Countdown: 264 Days

Tuesday, February 12, 2019

<u>Colorado Springs, CO</u>

I drink a cup of coffee to start the morning. I used to love coffee, drinking two cups every day with a total of 240 mg of caffeine. At the beginning of the year, I started tapering down on coffee consumption after learning that coffee may raise cholesterol even though it does have anti-inflammatory and antioxidant properties. In January, I signed up for and began studying the online Plant-Based Nutrition Course from eCornell University. It has been an amazing journey with students from all over the world, eager to learn about whole food plant-based nutrition. I am awed by our incredible and complex bodies and also their simplicity. My philosophy is to put only beneficial substances into my sacred body. What we feed our body has direct results on how we feel, both physically and emotionally. I am learning about the tremendous impact of nutrition.

I drink green tea in the morning and today the tea seems to provide only hydration without the effects of caffeine. I prefer a hot drink, and most of the time I will make my hot drink with ginger, turmeric, cacao, black pepper, and a hint of honey. This has become my favorite after-workout drink.

My energy is low this morning, so I decide to drink coffee and kick off the morning with qigong. I love qigong. I can do it anywhere without a yoga mat or a yoga outfit. I can simply do qigong sitting at my desk. Just breathing deeply puts me in harmony and balance. Ten minutes of morning qigong puts me in a state of clarity and intention for the day. I plan to offer qigong to my lifestyle coaching clients and Airbnb guests. This is a wonderful before-breakfast tool to wake the body with calm and balanced energy.

Countdown: 263 Days
Wednesday, February 13, 2019
Colorado Springs, CO

I should title this journal entry "Against the wind in both directions." I went out for a tempo run this morning and it was all about the wind whipping at my face and battering me from all sides. With every step I took, the wind pushed me in another direction. Nature is teaching me to be resilient. Okay, I get it, training in harsh conditions can be beneficial even though I don't enjoy it at the time. Nevertheless, I finished today's planned training. I rarely cheat and cut the training short. My coach creates my personalized schedule for successful marathon runs. My job is to follow it.

Countdown: 262 Days
Thursday, February 14, 2019
Colorado Springs, CO

The wind has continued blowing, with wind gusts up to 40 mph this morning, and I'm scheduled to run eight miles. The weather forecast shows the wind dying down later in the afternoon and I have a dilemma. Should I run inside on the treadmill, wait until this afternoon to run, or go outside now and be blown away by the wind? The treadmill seems like a safe bet and I head to the gym after eating the Valentine's Day breakfast Craig prepared. Breakfast came complete with a beautiful card as Craig always makes a homemade card with favorite photos and thoughtful words. This Valentine's Day was no exception.

As I said before and will again, we have an amazing relationship and are both very fortunate to love, live with, and appreciate each other. Craig and I are both taking our relationship to the next level through love, caring, and compassion. This afternoon Craig surprised me with a dozen red roses and then we had a couple's massage which was so warm and relaxing that I almost fell asleep. Craig prepared a special dinner, Hot Louisiana Style Soy Curls, from Michael Greger's "How Not to Die Cookbook." After dinner, we watched a movie, "The Eternal Sunshine of the Spotless Mind." It was indeed a special day.

Countdown: 261 Days

Friday, February 15, 2019

<u>Colorado Springs, CO</u>

I jogged two miles to the gym this morning to do my strength training. Craig and his friend, GW, are running/jogging up to Barr Camp this morning; Craig left at 6:40 to meet GW at Memorial Park in Manitou Springs at 7:00. I used to run/jog up to Barr Camp with Craig but, nowadays, Craig and I have different workout purposes and are out of sync in our training schedules. I enjoy the Manitou Incline. No matter how fit you are or how many times you have climbed it, the Incline will test you every time. My best Incline time is 38 minutes. Any workout pain is erased from my memory after reaching the top and looking down at the city.

The Incline is world-famous for its beautiful views from the top and steep 45% average grade as it gains over 2,000 vertical feet (610 m) of elevation up 2,768 railroad tie steps—the remnants of a 0.8-mile cable car route up the side of the mountain and a great workout by itself. From the top of the Incline, it's another four miles to Barr Camp, a rustic bed and breakfast at 10,200 feet (3,109 m) elevation. We appreciate and enjoy both the full-time and part-time caretakers who live there. They are always pleasant and eager to give us the weather conditions at the top of Pikes Peak along with their latest running stories. One of the caretakers is a world-class ultra-distance mountain trail racer, Zack Miller. He moved from Pennsylvania, lives at Barr Camp, and trains on the surrounding trails. He wins races all over the world. Jonathan is another amazing caretaker. He also races trails and roads. Regan, a young woman from Kansas, is also a runner. All three are amazing people living their dreams in a very unique way.

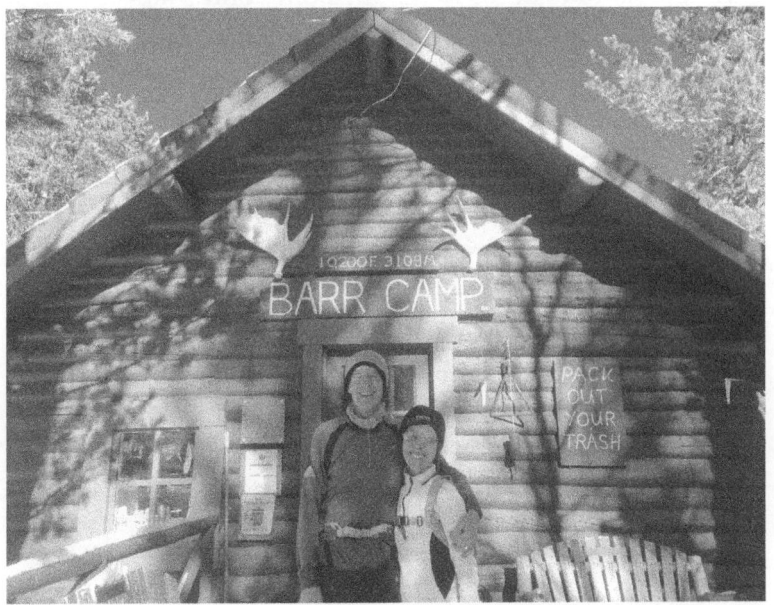

Barr Camp

Countdown: 260 Days

Saturday, February 16, 2019

Colorado Springs, CO

After two days of horrendous gusts, the wind finally subsided. It is a gorgeous, overcast Saturday morning, perfect for my 16-mile run. After eating my usual pre-run breakfast, I grab the energy drink I prepared the previous evening, and am out the door at 6:40. My energy drink consists of four Medjool dates, one tablespoon of peanut butter, one tablespoon of cacao, a half-inch each of finely grated turmeric root and ginger root, and eight ounces of water. I blend all the ingredients together in a Blendtec blender. It's delicious and gives me energy on my long runs.

Today, I am running on the Santa Fe Trail. The Woodmen trailhead is four miles from our home and this is my first time on the Santa Fe trail this year. The Santa Fe Trail is a well-maintained 8- to 10-foot-wide gravel trail with plenty of room for both bikers and runners, though today, a few spots on the trail are covered with sheet ice. The trail meanders through the US Air Force Academy and I am almost to the North Gate entrance of the Academy when I hear cars on I-25 zipping by. I focus my gaze on the snow-covered mountains bordering the west side of the Academy. It seems that today is a training day for everyone. I see so many young runners passing by me like a fast train. I pass a few runners in my age group and they stop and cheer me on saying "Good job," or "Keep going." I soak in the encouragement and finish my 16-mile run at an 11:06 minute/mile pace. Yay!

Countdown: 258 Days
Monday, February 18, 2019
<u>Colorado Springs, CO</u>

I wake up to four inches of snow on the ground and a temperature in the single digits. My training schedule today calls for hill repeats. We live in the Piñon Valley subdivision and right off the neighborhood park, we have "Steep Mother" hill—a constant slope gravel road leading uphill into Ute Valley Park, a wooded park crisscrossed with single-track trails. I usually do my hill repeats on Steep Mother. It's frigid out today and I decide to do my hill repeats on the treadmill at the gym. Craig suggests a six to seven percent grade for 90 seconds with a 2-minute, zero-percent grade cooldown between "hills." I do eight repeats and then continue to run for a total of 6.35 miles. Whew, that was 60 minutes of fun. I am about to finish when my running friend, Rod, steps onto a treadmill next to me and gives me a high five. He is a fast runner but lately has been battling health issues. Even during chemotherapy, though, he was logging 45+ miles per week. He is an amazingly strong runner and I suspect his running helps combat his health issues. Perhaps he forgets about his troubles when he is running. Whatever the reason, I hope he is listening to his body.

Countdown: 257 Days
Tuesday, February 19, 2019
Colorado Springs, CO

I'm glad I picked up and read a book titled, "Meb for Mortals," by Meb Keflezighi, a book on how to train, think, and eat. The most valuable lessons I acquired from the book were focusing on stretching and cross-training. I do cross-training exercises three days a week and yoga twice a week as part of my training. As Meb states, "It is not rehab, it's prehab."

Countdown: 256 Days
Wednesday, February 20, 2019
Colorado Springs, CO

I run intervals on the treadmill again today since the trails are covered with snow and ice, and the temperature is in the teens. I run at an 8-minute/mile pace for a half-mile with a half-mile recovery between intervals at a 9.5-minute/mile pace. I repeat these intervals for 60 minutes and finish with a total distance of 6.35 miles.

Countdown: 255 Days
Thursday, February 21, 2019
Colorado Springs, CO

I leave the house at 6:15 a.m. in the dark for today's 12-mile run. The trails are covered with snow and ice from yesterday's snowstorm. It's a cold 15°F, but there's no wind. I run up Flying W Ranch Road, about one mile of steep uphill. When I reach the top of the hill, I am out of breath, but I know if there is an uphill there must be a downhill to look forward to. I run down the hill to 30th Street and then turn around for another uphill climb and downhill descent. The total run is 9.3 miles.

At home, I eat two pancakes before running 2.15 miles to the Rockrimmon Library for a meeting with my Toastmaster mentee. She is preparing for the club-level International Speech contest and wants me to review her speech. Her speech content is solid, and I suggest she organize her speech in a slightly different sequence to smooth out the flow. I also recommend she plug in a few take-away nuggets in the beginning, during the body, and at the end of the speech. She wants to meet again on Monday after she incorporates my suggestions. I run home for a total of 13.6 miles for the day and feel good about my long-run training day. I've read several opinions on the effectiveness of splitting up a long run into multiple runs during the day. My understanding is that it all depends on the individual, the individual's schedule, and his/her ability. I'm not a professional athlete or an athletic coach, so I believe that listening to my own body furnishes the best answer for me.

Countdown: 254 Days
Friday, February 22, 2019
<u>Colorado Springs, CO</u>

As I look at the beautiful snow-covered mountains just across the valley from our home, I feel fortunate to be living in Colorado Springs. Training for a spring marathon is no small undertaking when living in a cooler part of the US and especially when we are experiencing our "best" (i.e., snowiest) winter in many years. We do have abundant sunshine though, with occasional bitter wind and icy trails. Today I am scheduled for strength training at the gym in anticipation of tomorrow's 20k race, the Winter Series IV race at the Penrose Event Center in Bear Creek Park.

Countdown: 253 Days
Saturday, February 23, 2019
<u>Colorado Springs, CO</u>

At 8:44 it is 25°F and sunny at the Norris Penrose Event Center where the Winter Series IV race is taking place. The race starts at 10:00, but I arrive early with Craig who is working as a car-parking volunteer for the race. It snowed six inches overnight and the mountain peaks are covered in white. The race trail is covered with snow. I warm up in the car with my energy drink, banana, and water, trying to eat something a couple of hours before the race start.

I know it will be slow going in the snow, but faster runners will pack down the snow for slower runners. My prediction is right. When the race starts, runners become congested into a single packed-down track and are barely moving. The first mile is very slow before we climb to the Mike Shafai memorial bench, sponsored by the Sunrise Striders, at the top of the hill. Mike was a pillar of the Colorado Springs running community. I admired Mike's attitude, kindness, and enthusiasm for life. Unfortunately, the finish line for Mike came unexpectedly and way too soon. The entire running community mourned his sudden loss a year and a half ago. I attended his funeral. It was beautiful and I couldn't help the sorrowful flow of tears. For all of us runners, there will be a finish line coinciding with the end of our running career. So, I say we should enjoy running while we are able. I yell out to Mike, "We miss you," and I see his face with a big smile replying "Hae, pick up the pace." His optimism, enthusiasm, and positive energy push me up the hill. I am so grateful for the opportunity to compete, something I could not have written about in my book ten years ago. I had a great race in the snow with a 10:21 minute/mile pace and came in second place in my age group.

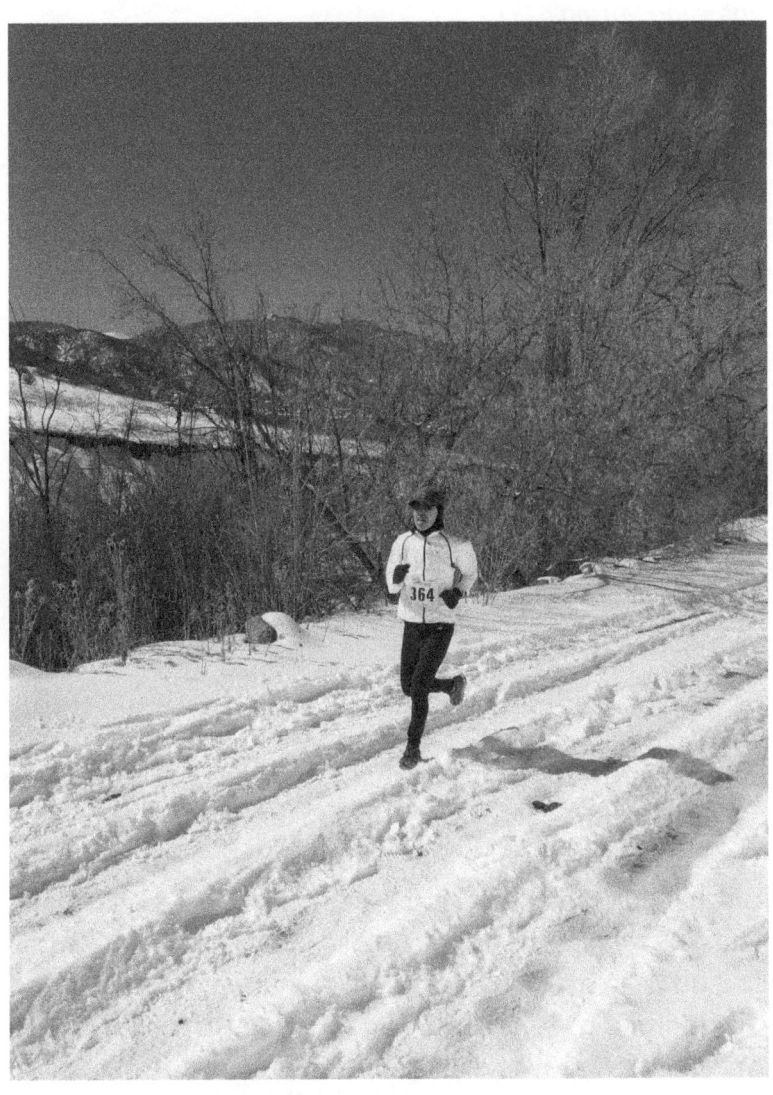

Hae Running in the Winter Series IV Race

Countdown: 252 Days

Sunday, February 24, 2019

<u>Colorado Springs, CO</u>

 I slept in this morning and did a strength workout at the gym. It's a beautiful day with the snow nearly melted and residual icy spots in the shady areas. We have a hectic schedule going into the week, so I decide to help Craig out with the grocery shopping for the second time this month. He's excited that I'm joining him and as I push the shopping cart and stock up on fruit, greens, veggies, sweet potatoes, avocados, berries, and other foods we love, he grabs a little sample cup of coffee with a big smile on his face. It's a lucky day for Craig.

Countdown: 251 Days

Monday, February 25, 2019

<u>Colorado Springs, CO</u>

 I am back to hill repeats on Steep Mother. The entrance hill into Ute Valley Park is covered with snow and ice, but I see a couple of gravel strips where people have been walking. Okay, that's the path I'll run up and come back down on. On the way up, I run into Steve, our neighbor, and his dog, Riley. Craig and I see Steve on Tuesday and Thursday evenings at yoga class. Steve warns me to be careful as there are a lot of icy spots on the trail and I thank him for his heads up. I also run into young runners wearing shorts in the 20-degree temperature. They are going up the hill while I am coming down. I give them high fives and continue down. I run eight hill repeats and finish with a cool-down run for a total of 6.35 fantastic miles this morning.

Countdown: 250 Days

Tuesday, February 26, 2019

<u>Colorado Springs, CO</u>

It is 25°F and sunny for today's run. Although this is my strength training day, I've decided to run instead. This will get me in sync with Craig's running schedule as we've been out of sync for most of the week. Also, tomorrow we have a Toastmasters meeting ending at 8:00 which is a bit later than I prefer for running. I love to run first thing in the morning, usually after breakfast, especially if I'm doing a long run, but sometimes even before breakfast. It is so delightful to run without any pressure and a good way to start the day.

Countdown: 249 Days

Wednesday, February 27, 2019

<u>Colorado Springs, CO</u>

I love the moisture in the air this morning. It's almost misting, something we don't frequently experience in this dry Colorado clime. I'm awed by the many types of weather we get in Colorado Springs—wind, sun, snow, rain, and hail. None of it stays around for long except for the sunny days. There's even a saying in Colorado, "If you don't like the weather, wait five minutes." March is just around the corner, and spring can be volatile here in the Rockies. I'm sure I will experience all the elements of weather next month.

Countdown: 248 Days

Thursday, February 28, 2019

<u>Colorado Springs, CO</u>

It is 6:45, calm and in the 30s as I start my 18-mile Boston Marathon profile training run. I run down Sinton Trail to the Pikes Peak Greenway Trail which then connects to the Santa Fe trail. I run home via Woodman Road for a total of 19.5 miles. I ran out of my 8-ounce energy drink at mile16, which teaches me that either I started consuming it too soon or I need to make more to get through the last six miles in a marathon. This is a good learning experience before the marathon. At least I still had plenty of water left over in my 32-ounce CamelBak bladder.

This is the first long training run in preparation for the Boston Marathon and I have only six more weeks of training. While I'm on the trail, I keep asking myself, "Why am I doing this?" and the answer is not easy. I'm not a natural-born runner and I didn't acquire long-running legs from my parents (they were both short with short legs). I was born and raised in Korea to Korean parents. Korean is my first language and all my siblings still live in Korea. No one in my family knows anything about running and my sisters keep saying I'm crazy to put such a burden on my body. I've stopped telling them about my running because their answer will always be the same, "You are crazy." I find running meditative and hope someday to find a clear and confident answer to the "why."

I see college kids on the trail today. They pass me like fast cars on a racetrack. I'm glad I didn't start out running in high school, not that it was an option for me. There were no running programs and no college scholarships for running. The only running I had to perform was for the high school entrance requirement, a 400m run to check off the box on the school enrollment document. At the end of the 400m run, I passed out. Luckily, I'd completed the 400m and got into high school anyway!

I graduated high school second in my class of 600 students. This was a big Korean high school and my boyfriend graduated first in our class. During the weekends, my boyfriend and I hung out and worked out solutions to geometry and calculus problems. Sports of any kind were not in my blood. I was a bookworm who excelled at academics and went on to complete a college degree. You might say I was a late bloomer. I didn't even start running until the age of 55 after my first husband passed away. Running gave me a sense of my time with nature and the meditation eased my sorrow and heartbreak. Eventually, I met Craig. He had been running for many years and I started training with him. The very first race I signed up for was the 50-mile Run Rabbit Run ultra-marathon in high-altitude Steamboat Springs, Colorado. When I signed up, I didn't fully realize the training commitment necessary to complete a 50-mile run. With Craig's fantastic hands-off coaching style, we both finished the 50-mile race. The race allowed me to realize that I could be a runner. That's where it all began.

I love having a race goal and progressing toward it. Without targeted goals, it would still be fun to be out there running, but specific goals give me more focus. I am all about making progress every day, every workout, every speech I give, and every client I coach. Progress is "success," no matter how small. And maybe that's the answer to my "why" question. Progress through process. It's not the end game that is most important, it's all about making progress and having fun doing it. No one gives two cents about your personal record (PR), or your finish place in local races. But, for me, appreciating and having fun with the process of reaching my goal is the most important thing. And running keeps me healthy, sharp, and happy mentally and physically. I'm glad I was able to answer my "why" question by the end of today's long run.

Countdown: 247 Days
Friday, March 1, 2019
<u>Colorado Springs, CO</u>

Wow, March already. Time is flying by and I only have a few more weeks until the Boston Marathon. Today, I'm doing strength training at the gym. I don't feel any negative aftereffects from yesterday's long run. Amazing.

We had our running friend, Rod, and his wife, Alisa, over for a pasta dinner. I have never met anyone with so many interesting stories, starting from his childhood in Boy Scouts through his military service, his running, and his job. It's 9:30 p.m., already an hour past my bedtime, and Rod is still talking. When I look over at Craig, his eyes are half-closed. I'm also tired and I have a speed workout scheduled in the morning. I get up and clear the dinner table to give Rod and Alisa a hint that it's time to wrap up the evening. It was a fun evening though, and I'm impressed that he is both a remarkable runner and has had such an interesting life.

Countdown: 246 Days
Saturday, March 2, 2019
Colorado Springs, CO

Craig and I are playing hooky from our Toastmasters District Officer Training in Longmont, a little over two hours north of Colorado Springs. We sent out a request to the universe to send us some snow so we didn't have to attend the training meeting, and the universe delivered. It's snowing in Longmont and snow will be arriving in Colorado Springs this afternoon.

It's not that I don't want the training, it's just that it is such a long drive. I'd rather be out running than sitting in a car for two hours each way. Craig and I are both Toastmaster Area Directors, which means we each have four clubs to oversee in our respective areas. It's fun to visit the other clubs and observe how they conduct meetings and to help them with their challenges. At the same time, it's a lot of effort to visit clubs and submit reports to Toastmasters International. It would make the training easier if Toastmasters International would adopt video conferencing, minimizing absenteeism due to weather and allowing online training to avoid travel.

Instead of spending the day in a car and a classroom, I did my scheduled speed workout. It was a perfect morning for it, and I encountered several other runners on the trail. I purchased lightweight, 5.75-ounce, Altra brand "Boston" shoes and am trying them out today. I love how light my feet feel, as though they are weightless with every step.

Countdown: 245 Days
Sunday, March 3, 2019

<u>Colorado Springs, CO</u>

It's a lovely day with big snowflakes continuously falling. Already, several inches of snow have accumulated. Luckily, today is my gym strength training day. I love my gym, especially the sauna, on days like today. I soak in the heat and meditate while sweat is coming out of my pores like little fountains of water.

I have seen snow like this in Maine where I lived for 20 years and raised my kids. After my two children graduated from college and got their own places, my first husband and I decided to explore the West. We flew out to Utah and visited Snowbird Ski Resort. We fell in love with Utah. So much so, that we sold our house in Maine and purchased a townhome in Park City, Utah. Today's snow reminds me of Park City.

During our first year in Utah, Alex, my son, Mira, my daughter, and Pete, Mira's significant other, joined us for a ski vacation at Brighton Ski Resort. The snow was coming down so hard that the road up Little Cottonwood Canyon to Snowbird was closed due to avalanche danger. Since Big Cottonwood Canyon road was open, we drove to Brighton Ski Resort. When we made it out for our first run, the snow was coming down so hard I got buried in the powder and couldn't even ski. All the expert skiers in the family—my first husband, Chris, plus Alex, Mira, and Pete were in heaven, hopping through the powder like ski bunnies. It was so much fun.

Nowadays, Craig and I ski five days on a good year and zero to one on a Boston marathon training year. The drive from Colorado Springs to the closest ski area, Breckenridge, is over two hours. When we go skiing, we like to stay overnight near the ski area, since a four-hour drive is too much for a half-day of skiing. Craig and I had season passes and skied a lot when we dated and lived together in Park City. Three ski areas, Canyons, Park City, and Deer Valley were all within a 15-minute drive. We could sleep in until 7:00, have breakfast, and still get to the mountain by 9:00. Somedays, we went out for only a couple of hours of skiing. Craig and his skiing friends were competing to see who would ski the most days for the season. One of Craig's friends, Joel, won the competition, skiing for more than 45 days. He would go almost every day, even if for only one run, just to say he skied. Fun times.

Countdown: 244 Days

Monday, March 4, 2019

Colorado Springs, CO

It snowed 10 inches overnight and hill repeats are on the training schedule this morning. I love snow but not on a hill repeat day, because I can't tell where the ice patches are hiding under the fluffy white stuff. Safety is number one on my list, so I'm hitting the gym this morning. I set the treadmill at an eight percent incline for the 90-second uphills and a zero-degree incline for the 60-second cooldown between each hill. I do 10 hill repeats and complete one hour of running for a total of 6.3 miles. Excellent workout.

Countdown: 243 Days

Tuesday, March 5, 2019

<u>Colorado Springs, CO</u>

It's a white winter wonderland out this morning with the thermometer showing only 8°F. All the trees are covered with snow. The pine trees are especially beautiful as I run by on the Foothills Trail, an eight-foot-wide pea-gravel and snow-plowed trail. I love pine trees. They're green all year, and I especially love them in the winter as they stand fully clothed when the deciduous trees are naked, having dropped all their leaves. I tiptoe over the longer icy patches and hop over the smaller icy spots, landing on dry trail.

My calendar is open today. After the run and cleaning up, I will have a couple of pancakes and then meditate. Craig and I will be attending a Toastmasters International Speech Contest in the evening at the Cheyenne Mountain Library, one of the many branch libraries of the Pikes Peak Library District. We'll be supporting Greg and Mary T. who are representing our Pikes Peak Toastmasters club at the area contest. I am cheering for Mary T., my mentee. I have been helping her with her speech for several weeks. I hope she wins the contest and moves up to the division contest. (Although Mary T. gave a brilliant speech, another competitor won and will move up).

Countdown: 242 Days

Wednesday, March 6, 2019

<u>Colorado Springs, CO</u>

Our guest, Sarissa, left today after staying with us for five days. She was our Airbnb guest in 2018 and we invited her to stay with us while she attended an exercise training class this week to help Parkinson's disease patients. Sarrisa exudes enthusiasm with everything she does, and her enthusiasm brightens our lives. It's a characteristic everyone should strive for no matter what is happening in life. If you are going to train for a marathon, train with a smile on your face. Perhaps enthusiasm will improve your performance? I believe that being positive and zealous will make everything better. Chunking and marginal progress are key. Today I am doing two sets of each of the following:

- 15 repetitions of wide-leg squats
- 15 repetitions of thigh lunges
- 12 repetitions of shoulder upright rows
- 12 repetitions of dumbbell bent-over rows
- High leg-rise walking
- My additional gym exercise routines

Today I do 50% more than my usual workout.

Countdown: 241 Days
Thursday, March 7, 2019
<u>Colorado Springs, CO</u>

Finally, the temperature is in the 40s and I can reduce my upper body clothing layers from three to two. I feel so much lighter. The sun is shining with a slight breeze. I feel light and amazing during my long run. One thing though, I'll need to make sure my Garmin GPS watch is fully charged on marathon day. When I grabbed my Garmin this morning, it decided to go into protest mode, so instead of waiting for it to charge up or trying to fix it, I decided to run without it. I used the Strava app on my phone and it worked out great.

It has cool features, such as recording the elevation gain and loss for every mile, but I don't want to carry it during a marathon. I had a superb 13.9-mile training run today.

Countdown: 240 Days
Friday, March 8, 2019
<u>Colorado Springs, CO</u>

Back to the gym for strength training. The best parts of gym day are the sauna and the shower. Like me, many of the same people are there at the gym, day after day, doing their workout routines.

Countdown: 239 Days
Saturday, March 9, 2019
<u>Colorado Springs, CO</u>

I wake up at 5:00 to the sound of gale-force winds. The house shakes as if it is about to lift off of its foundation. I know I have a scheduled interval speed workout of eight half-mile repeats. I need an hour and a half to complete the workout with a 1.5-mile warmup and a 1.5-mile cooldown at the end of the workout. Also, Craig and I are conducting the Toastmasters International Southern Division Area 1 and Area 2 Evaluation and International Speech Contests starting at 10:00 so I need to get out the door for my workout by 5:45. I'm hoping the wind will die down, but I don't see that happening anytime soon. After eating my pre-run breakfast, and turning on my headlamp, I'm out the door.

As soon as I'm on the trail, dawn lights the sky and I store the headlamp in my windbreaker. The wind is whipping me from the left, from the right, head-on, and occasionally from the back, which gives me a push and reduces my interval time by a few seconds. Despite the wind, this is the best I've felt all season. It's a wonderful breakthrough, as I've been struggling with my speed and my body's responses to hard running lately. I self-monitor my breathing during every training run to determine how I respond to the workload. Today I am confident, and my body feels light. I do some hard running and feel great.

The Toastmasters contests were successful and went off without any hiccups. Craig did an outstanding job as contest chair. My role was the chief judge. The contest was an area-level competition and the winners will progress to the division contest, and those winners then move on to the district-level competition. Toastmasters International is an outstanding organization helping people learn and grow their communication and leadership skills. Organizing the contest was a lot of work, but I had fun and it's a growth experience in delegation, organization, communication, and leadership skills. Most importantly, I took away valuable, life-enhancing messages from the speeches.

Countdown: 238 Days
Sunday, March 10, 2019
Colorado Springs, CO

I spent a lazy Sunday morning ignoring the daylight savings time change and slept in, getting a much-needed rest. Craig left the house early to go skiing with his daughter and her boyfriend. I decided not to take any unnecessary risks with only five weeks until the Boston Marathon. As much as I love skiing, it's not my favorite sport and there's a minimum four-hour, round-trip drive to ski for only a few hours. Also, I would have had to get up super early. Today I'm enjoying "ME" time by having a delicious breakfast of oatmeal with berries and my one cup of coffee for the day that I enjoy so much. I usually drink water when I get up and enjoy my coffee with my meal or after breakfast. Later, I'll watch my favorite type of movie. Craig and I have different preferences in movies. He loves science fiction love stories and I like documentaries and heartwarming movies.

Countdown: 237 Days
Monday, March 11, 2019
Colorado Springs, CO

Finally, just when I was enjoying the dawn light for my early morning runs, the change to daylight savings time put me back into pre-dawn darkness and running with a headlamp! Today I run hill repeats at the Ute Valley Park entrance. In the dark I see a shadow moving, which gives me a start; but it's just a guy with a dog. At the top of the ascent, I am out of breath. I take a few deep breaths before I descend again. I run ten hill repeats and finish up with another three easy miles to complete today's training run.

Countdown: 236 Days
Tuesday, March 12, 2019
Colorado Springs, CO

I decide to run a "moderate length" run of seven miles today. Strength training at the gym is on my training schedule, but I tend to listen to my body and adjust accordingly. I've become my own coach in addition to having a training coach. I've try to learn as much as I can about running and have read eight running books since January. I often watch YouTube videos to help improve my performance. I'll do my strength training tomorrow and a 20-mile run on Thursday. When I did back-to-back Wednesday/Thursday long runs, it wasn't effective for me and my Thursday workout suffered. I modified my schedule to do hill repeats on Monday, a moderate run on Tuesday, strength training on Wednesday, my long run on Thursday, strength training on Friday, and my interval speed workout on Saturday.

Countdown: 235 Days
Wednesday, March 13, 2019
Colorado Springs, CO

Whiteout blizzard conditions with blowing snow are predicted for today. The schools and businesses have already shut down because of the winter storm forecast. It's going to be a gym and cross-training day. After my workout, I make it home before the first snowflake. The snowstorm hits shortly after we return home. Tomorrow isn't looking good for my 20-mile run. The trails will be covered with new and drifted snow and are bound to be slippery. I can't remember the last day I had ideal weather and trail conditions for training. I don't usually worry about things I don't have control over, and the weather is one of those things no one can control. I have to flow with whatever comes and adjust my training schedule accordingly. The forecast predicts that Saturday will have much better weather, so I tentatively plan to push my

20-mile run to Saturday but will make my final decision early tomorrow morning.

Countdown: 234 Days
Thursday, March 14, 2019
Colorado Springs, CO

I debate whether to do today's training run since yesterday's blizzard left us with ice and a foot of drifted snow. In the end, I decided to do a speed workout rather than try to navigate the snow-covered trail for my 20-mile run. I put traction on my shoes (cleats connected with chains held on to my shoes by an elastic band). I know it will slow me down, but safety is number one and I can't afford a fall on the ice. It is a brutal speed workout on the snow and ice, but I accomplished it despite the piercing wind, low air temperature, and cloud cover.

Countdown: 233 Days
Friday, March 15, 2019
Colorado Springs, CO

Today is strength training at the gym but my nose begins to run. I know my body well and make sage, lemon, and honey tea—my go-to drink when I feel something starting in my nose or throat. I hate being sick. My motto is pre-vention rather than post-vention. The morning after my cup of sage tea, I'm as good as new. I've shared my secret remedy with many friends, and it's worked like magic for them too.

Countdown: 232 Days

Saturday, March 16, 2019

Colorado Springs, CO

    Today I plan to run 20 miles. I head out at 6:30 just as the dawn light illuminates the horizon. I prefer to run without a headlamp, so this is the perfect time to begin my run. With the snow and ice from Wednesday's blizzard, I watch my steps. The asphalt in the short but narrow and dark tunnel under Centennial Boulevard is covered with windblown snow and ice. I carefully tiptoe through. The Pikes Peak Greenway Trail is plowed and clear, so I pick up the pace to the Santa Fe Trail entrance at Woodmen Road. Once again, the trail has not been plowed. It's enveloped in two feet of snow and ice. I recognize many familiar faces on the trail. I trudge forward two and a half miles through the deep snow and turn around at the 10-mile point. The trail is not runnable. I begin running again once I reach the Pikes Peak Greenway Trail, then continue running up Sinton Trail. Other than having to walk that snowy bit on the Santa Fe Trail, I completed my 20-mile run.

Countdown: 231 Days

Sunday, March 17, 2019

Colorado Springs, CO

    It is back to the gym for strength training. It's a great day to give my legs a rest from yesterday's long run and do some stretching. I'll also be giving my body a rest for tomorrow's hill repeats. While there, I talk to my running friend, Rod. Besides admiring him as a fast runner, I enjoy his many stories. I think he could talk for 24-hours without stopping. Some people have that talent (and life experience), and he is an amazing person and storyteller.

Countdown: 230 Days
Monday, March 18, 2019
Colorado Springs, CO

It's a pleasant, calm morning and the sun is ready to light up the top of Pikes Peak. From our dining room window, I have a clear view of the snow-covered peak. It's stunning when the morning sun hits the top of the mountain.

It's hill repeat day again. I love hill repeats for my legs, glutes, and lungs. They also teach me how to breathe. We start breathing when we are born, but it's when I'm running uphill that I learn how to breathe deeply. Later, my breathing returns to normal, moving air automatically in and out of my lungs 24-hours a day, facilitating the exchange of oxygen and carbon dioxide. We have the perfect training hill close to home and, as usual, my focus moves to my breathing and my legs. Today is my best time up the hill at 1 minute 32 seconds. My 10 hill repeats are all under 1 minute 38 seconds—my best so far this year.

Countdown: 229 Days
Tuesday, March 19, 2019
Colorado Springs, CO

It seems the wind is always blowing when I run, whether I go before or after sunrise. Also, it seems the wind is always blowing into my face! Again, I must surrender to the elements. Perhaps nature is trying to teach me to be a tougher runner with all she has to offer—wind, sun, cold, ice, snow, and rain. Today, I run one steep mile up Flying W Ranch Road. I run a 10:30 minute/mile pace up the hill, a new record for me. I'm finally getting into shape after some less-than-stellar January and February training runs. It's mid-March, with only a few weeks before the Boston Marathon, and I'm beginning to peak in my performance. I would like to be faster, though. My goal is to get my pace under 10 minutes/mile for long runs, although my coach says long runs should be one to two minutes per mile slower than race-day pace, so I guess I won't be pushing speed at this stage. I'm listening carefully to my body. Better to be slower and healthy during training than to never start or be unable to finish the marathon.

Countdown: 228 Days
Wednesday, March 20, 2019
Colorado Springs, CO

Bib#: 24764
Wave/Corral: 4/1
Name: Bolduc, Hae
Age: 63
M/F: F
City: Colorado Springs

I received my Boston Marathon bib Number and Corral assignment from the Boston Athletic Association. My heart is already pounding with nervousness and excitement in anticipation of the event. After another week and a half of training, I'll start my taper. I can't believe how fast it's coming. Today is a perfect day for a run and this is my speed workout day. I see my running friend, Rod, on the trail and he comments "Your legs show you have been putting some mileage in." Yes, I have been putting in some mileage along with hard workouts.

Countdown: 227 Days
Thursday, March 21, 2019
Colorado Springs, CO

    Twelve miles seems like an easy run these days compared to the 20-mile runs. It is the first time in a long time that I feel pretty good during my moderate distance run.

Countdown: 226 Days
Friday, March 22, 2019
Colorado Springs, CO

    My client is on vacation in the Caribbean, so I'm taking advantage of my free time from my life-coaching session and go to the gym with Craig. He loves Friday gym workouts after Thursday's long Barr Camp run. For a couple of hours, he works hard on his upper body and stretches. He isn't planning to run any races this year but works as hard as if he'll be racing next week. I love that his habits and discipline are so ingrained.

Countdown: 225 Days
Saturday, March 23, 2019
<u>Manitou Springs, CO</u>

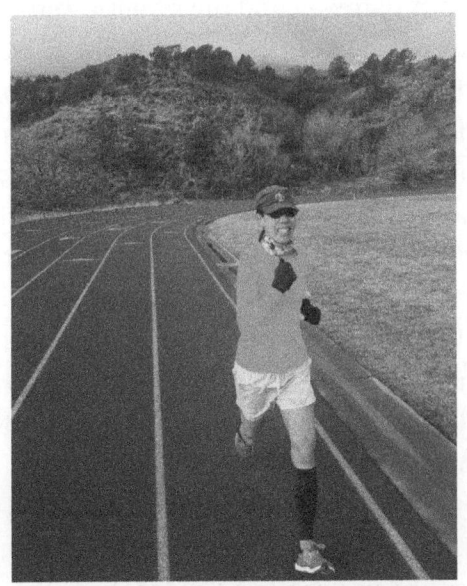

Manitou Springs High School Track

My coach and I are heading to the fast and rubberized Manitou Springs High School Track, which is open to the public. It's a beautiful location with Pikes Peak in the background. He has me do a slow 1-mile warmup followed by fast 6x800m intervals with slow 400m recovery runs in between the intervals. The sky is overcast with the temperature in the 30s and no wind. Perfect conditions for my interval workout. I run 3:57 for the first 800m, then slow to 4:10 - 4:17 for the remaining 800s.

Countdown: 224 Days

Sunday, March 24, 2019

Rye, CO

Today is our date day and my sweetie and I are heading south to visit Bishop Castle. We make the drive of an hour and a half from our home after doing strength training at the gym. I prefer not to be sitting in a car for that length of time, but the weather is good for driving, so we pack our lunch and head down to Rye, Colorado. Jim Bishop started building the Castle over 60 years ago and construction has continued ever since. The architecture vaguely reminds me of Sagrada Familia in Barcelona Spain, a huge, unfinished Roman Catholic church. Construction of the Sagrada Familia began in 1882, and starting in 1883 the architecture was guided by Antoni Gaudí until he died in 1926. The church construction continues today, just as construction on Bishop Castle continues today. It would be fun to see the completion of the project, but I suspect construction of the castle will continue long after Bishop is gone. For me, I'd want to see the completion of a lifelong project. I'm glad that marathons have a beginning and an end. It gives me a sense of accomplishment and closure no matter the outcome. I'm already nervous about winding down my training after this week's 20-mile run and I look forward to finishing the race with a sense of closure for my hard labor.

Countdown: 223 Days

Monday, March 25, 2019

Colorado Springs, CO

Back to 10x hill repeats. Hill workouts are the best for building strength in my legs, glutes, and heart. I love

Steep Mother. It's wonderful living so close to such perfect locations for all my workouts—hill repeats (Ute Valley Park entrance), hill climbs (Flying W Ranch Road—one mile ascent and descent), long runs (Sinton Trail connecting to Pikes Peak Greenway Trail, then to Santa Fe Trail), speed workouts (Manitou Springs High School Track). Got to love this city.

Countdown: 222 Days

Tuesday, March 26, 2019

Colorado Springs, CO

 I run a moderate seven mile distance over Flying W Ranch Road summit with steady uphill climbing and fast leg turnover during the descent. I turn around and return over the same hill. This is the first day this year I've run in shorts and calf compressors. I love the perfect, sunny, 39°F training weather. It is indeed an ideal spring training day.

Countdown: 221 Days

Wednesday, March 27, 2019

Colorado Springs, CO

 It's sunny and surprisingly warm with a high-temperature forecast of 70°F. It would feel wonderful to run and soak up the heat this morning, however, it's my gym day. My legs will need a break from running since I plan to do 20 miles tomorrow. Sometimes I just feel like going out for a run instead of sticking to a schedule, but I'll adhere to it through the marathon. Challenges are a part of life. They help us to grow and become resilient—necessary elements in life, even if it leaves us with an uneasy feeling when we face them. I believe that embracing challenges and overcoming difficulties leads us to realize our highest potential.

Countdown: 220 Days
Thursday, March 28, 2019
Colorado Springs, CO

    I start my long run at 6:00. It's already 50°F and I run in shorts and a lightweight long sleeve shirt. I also pack my windbreaker just in case. I run down Sinton Trail, connect to the Pikes Peak Greenway Trail, and then run north past Woodmen Road onto the Santa Fe Trail. There's a nice breeze as I run, and the overcast skies remind me of New England. After 15 miles I find that my 32-ounce water bladder is empty, and I run the last five miles without water. I feel pumped up to have run an average minute/mile pace of 10:02. It's a good pace and a good accomplishment for me. This was my final long training run before beginning my two-and-a-half-week taper for the Boston Marathon.

Countdown: 219 Days
Friday, March 29, 2019
Colorado Springs, CO

    I'm taking a nice, easy gym day after yesterday's long run. My legs feel unaffected by yesterday's run. Recovering quickly makes running enjoyable. I am truly astonished by how often I feel great the day after a long run. I believe that the way I treat my body has a lot to do with this. In addition to eating plant-based whole foods with no animal products—eggs, dairy, meat, or fish—I also meditate for 30 minutes after waking up around 5:00. My sleep routine is also key to taking care of myself. At 8:00 p.m. I'm ready to slow down and relax with a good book, which puts me into a quiet state of mind before dropping off to sleep.

Countdown: 218 Days
Saturday, March 30, 2019
Manitou Springs High School Track

I'm back at the Manitou Springs High School track for a speed-interval workout. It's cloudy and a bit windy with the temperature in the mid-20s and a couple of inches of new snow on the ground from last night's storm. This is my last interval training workout before the Boston Marathon. Yay! My track workout today is a "ladder." It consists of 4x400m, 2x800m, 1x1600m, 2x800m, and back down the ladder with 4x400m. I try to give it my all. I feel fast and my 400 meters clocks in at a pace of 1:58 minutes/mile, which makes me happy. Speed training is tough, but every time I finish, I feel wonderfully pumped up on endorphins.

Countdown: 217 Days
Sunday, March 31, 2019
Colorado Springs, CO

It's our date day. Craig is rents the movie "Touching the Void," which is an unbelievable story based on true events in 1987 on the Siula Grande mountain in the Peruvian Andes. Two young British climbers set out to ascend Siula Grande, but both faced different and horrifying ordeals, including each believing that the other had died, and the challenges of facing their own deaths. Both survive through determination, perseverance, and strong will.

Oh my gosh, I think running 26.2 miles is difficult. Well, yes, it is, but what these two climbers went through is like facing the last six miles in a marathon continuously for seven horrific days. I guess when I run the Boston Marathon and hit the wall late in the race, I can think about the resilience and grit of these two climbers to help me push through to the finish line.

Countdown: 216 Days
Monday, April 1, 2019
<u>*Colorado Springs, CO*</u>

Wow, it's April! I've entered the month of the 2019 Boston Marathon and there are only two weeks to go until the race. I'm a bit restless and unsettled this morning. My coach has me starting my two-week taper, meaning that I will decrease my running quantity to be completely rested and twitching with energy on marathon day. I did my last hill repeats (6x) this morning, knowing that I need to finish my training strong. My body has responded so well to my training that I feel like I can run forever, but I need to listen to my coach. I hear well, but usually follow the beat of my own drums. I like to do things my way, even if wrong, and learn from my mistakes.

I can't count all the mistakes I have made in my life's journey. I'm sure I'll continue to make them but will hope for fewer as I move forward with my accumulated life wisdom. Can a human being ever reach a perfect state? And what is the meaning of "perfect?" According to the dictionary definition it is "having all the required or desirable elements, qualities, or characteristics; as good as it is possible to be."

Seeking perfection is something we have to pursue ourselves, in our own way, based on our own goals, and not something we can let others guide or choose for us.

Countdown: 215 Days

Tuesday, April 2, 2019

Colorado Springs, CO

I went out for a short 5-mile taper run this morning. I'm feeling great and hopefully, I'll still feel at the top of my running game on marathon day. There are always unknowns, however, including the weather and there's no way to predict how I'll feel come race day. Worrying doesn't help, though, so for now, I'll just try my best to live in the present and not worry about what marathon day will bring.

Countdown: 214 Days

Wednesday, April 3, 2019

Colorado Springs, CO

I do a total body workout for my core, upper body, legs, and hips at the gym today.

Countdown: 213 Days

Thursday, April 4, 2019

Colorado Springs, CO

I run my regular 8-mile Flying W Ranch Road route, climbing up to Mountain Shadows Pass and then descending to 30th Street, turning around and returning home the same way, up and down. It's a grueling route and I don't want to push too hard this close to the marathon. Regardless, I have a stupendous run. My usual ascent pace is 11:00 minutes/mile but today my pace is 10:25 minutes/mile. Wow. I'm feeling really strong on hill climbs now. I have improved in all areas of my training and feel I'm peaking in performance at just the right time. Progress, or more specifically, improvement is the key to everything we do in life. Without it, we are stagnating or heading in the wrong direction. No matter what we do, we want to progress, which I equate to "success." This is the same philosophy I use with my lifestyle coaching clients. Progress is "success."

Countdown: 212 Days
Friday, April 5, 2019
Colorado Springs, CO

Since my client canceled our coaching session this morning, I have spare time to work on our website, www.integratedlifestyletransformation.com. I know it's a long domain name and that the first advice someone would give is, "Use a shorter name," but we decided to use one that expresses our philosophy. We set up our website with WordPress and I love that our name reflects the theme of transformation. Our website was built by our friend, Steve, who we met as our Airbnb guest while he attended a three-day conference in Woodland Park. He is a generous person with a life philosophy of giving back to others.

After Steve built our website, I took over the maintenance, learning WordPress and helping the website evolve. I created a blog page and have posted several educational articles written by Craig: "Fit versus Healthy,"

"Food for Thought," and "Holistic Health Retreat Airbnb." I love Craig's writing style. Sometimes I get lost in his words and have to spend time in the online dictionary. A great benefit of managing the website is that I'm always learning new words as well as learning about WordPress and websites. English is a difficult second language to learn and, for me, I'll be continuing to work toward mastering it my entire lifetime.

Countdown: 211 Days
Saturday, April 6, 2019
<u>Colorado Springs, CO</u>

It's 6:20 and just before sunrise. The weather is ideal for my 6-mile run. This will be my last training run. Next week I'll just do short shakeout runs of three to four miles. It's hard to believe my hard training runs are over. Best of all, I feel so much stronger than I did at the beginning of the year. It's amazing how we adapt not only to hard training but also the wide variety of weather and other conditions. Honestly, I can count only a handful of days when the weather and trail conditions were ideal. The weather for 90% of my training days has been pretty brutal. I look back now with awe that I was out running in all those vicious conditions. After all that, I'm ready to go out and have fun at the marathon while soaking up the high energy of runners from around the world.

Countdown: 210 Days
Sunday, April 7, 2019

Colorado Springs, CO

The weather is gorgeous with irises and daylilies popping up from their winter sleep. Other plants, including weeds and grass, are also waking up and painting the brown and reddish winter ground with the green colors of spring. I'm enjoying the day after this morning's strength training at the gym followed by baking cacao energy bars for my pre-marathon snack. The energy bars contain oats, dates, cacao, almonds, and cherries. They taste like delicious chocolate cherry cake. I've been using this snack during my training runs and know that I handle the pre-race energy well. I'll be freezing some to take to Boston with me.

Countdown: 209 Days
Monday, April 8, 2019

Colorado Springs, CO

Unbelievable... it's only a week until the Boston Marathon. Here, it's another stunning spring day with temperatures in the 70s. At 7:00 it's already 50°F. The sun came up half an hour ago and it is a glorious day for a 4-mile run. I have only a couple of runs left before the marathon. This week I won't be doing anything new with exercise or nutrition. I will stay the course with what's familiar from the last three months of training.

Countdown: 208 Days

Tuesday, April 9, 2019

<u>Colorado Springs, CO</u>

I don't even remember the last time I ran JUST three miles. My route is mostly a rocky trail with tree stumps and uneven surfaces. I look ahead on the trail to make sure I don't trip and wipe out. I've fallen plenty of times and have gravity tattoos on my right and left knees to prove it. Craig is the one who refers to the scars as gravity tattoos. It sounds sexier than "running scars."

In 2013 I was training for the Steamboat Springs Run Rabbit Run 50-Mile Race. Craig and I were completing a 26-mile training run up Pikes Peak to Elk Park and back down. Almost back, I was within a couple of miles of the trailhead on Long's Ranch Road, in a very steep and slippery gravel section of the road called Papa Bear Hill. I was tired and running downhill too fast to control myself. I wiped out and slid down on my hands and knees. Looking at my bleeding knees, I was so upset that I told Craig, "Running is too dangerous. I will never run again." Quickly, my knees and hands healed, complete with gravity tattoos, and my drive to run returned. Craig and I ended up finishing the Run Rabbit Run 50-Mile Race in 13 hours 11 minutes 20 seconds.

Place: 117
Bib#: 1293
Name: Hae Bolduc
Elapsed: 13:11:20
Gender: F
Age: 57

Countdown: 207 Days

Wednesday, April 10, 2019

<u>Colorado Springs, CO</u>

Today is gym and Toastmaster meeting day. I won the Best Evaluator ribbon at our meeting this morning. Craig delivered a really fun speech on a research project taking us back in time to the 1950s, using the tobacco disease analogy to the current standard American disease diet. In the 1950s, doctors were smoking and the advertisements at the time promoted the cigarette brand "preferred by doctors." Today, doctors are eating everything on the market with little thought of the long-term consequences. I wondered how many people in the audience really got his message. Having extensively researched the causes of chronic diseases, Craig is passionate about educating people about a healthy lifestyle founded on eating plant-based whole food, exercise, meditation, and giving back to the community. Educating and inspiring people about a healthy lifestyle is difficult after a lifetime of negative conditioning and unquestioned false information. In the runners' world, many runners believe that because they are exercising and look fit, they are healthy and can eat anything. How faulty is that thinking?

Countdown: 206 Days

Thursday, April 11, 2019

<u>Colorado Springs, CO</u>

I ran an easy three miles this morning. After the 70° weather yesterday, it felt very cold with wind and the temperature in the 20s. My body was only just beginning to warm up by the end of the run.

Countdown: 205 Days

Friday, April 12, 2019

<u>Colorado Springs, CO</u>

I sent the following letter out today:

Dear Family and Friends,

It feels like an insurmountable task for me to run this historical 123rd Boston Marathon on April 15, 2019! I am truly grateful and am extremely emotional about the opportunity to run on my home turf, New England! It has been an audacious journey for me to tackle the training schedule my coach put together for the event. The hard training began in earnest at the beginning of 2019 in wintery snow, wind, ice, and cold; these conditions have strengthened and helped prepare me for this event. The Boston Marathon will test my endurance and perseverance to the maximum.

You can cheer me on—wherever you are, whatever you are doing—on April 15th, and push me to the finish line!

Thank you!

Name: Hae Bolduc
Bib Number: 24764

Download the Boston Marathon app
<u>http://live.sporthive.com/event/5512/app</u>

Countdown: 204 Days

Saturday, April 13, 2019

<u>Colorado Springs, CO</u>

I woke up early, mediated, and had my usual delicious oatmeal-blueberry pancakes with fruit and green tea. I won't drink coffee this morning. I have curbed my coffee consumption since Wednesday, and I won't drink it again until the morning of the race. I plan to cleanse coffee out of my system for five days and then drink it on race day for a performance boost. If you are a daily coffee drinker, then you need coffee just to get to your normal operating level. But if you metabolize it out of your body for a minimum of three days, the coffee can enhance your athletic performance. The weather forecast on race day is calling for some moisture, but I plan to bring sunshine from Colorado. I'm going to focus on the thought that it will be a great day for running. However, it's always a good idea to hope for the best and prepare for the worst, so that'll be my race day attire packing strategy.

As I review the "to take" list, it starts to feel real that the trip I've been anticipating for so long is actually here. The flight from Denver to Boston leaves at 3:45 p.m. which gives us all morning to get ready. It's snowing lightly as we prepare. When Craig left the house for his run, he reminded me, "No run for you today." He returned from his 5-mile run with a frozen bandana, windbreaker, and pants, fooled by the weather. He'd started his run in a light mist which quickly turned into a freezing mist.

Craig shows me the list of Colorado Springs runners who are signed up for the Boston Marathon; there are over 50, including a few elite runners. I'm proud to be among them.

Countdown: 203 Days

Sunday, April 14, 2019

<u>Somerville, MA</u>

    We arrived late last night at our Airbnb in Somerville, Massachusetts. When Craig made the reservations, he said the place was 0.7 miles away from a Red Line subway station. I had a hard time sleeping because of street noise. The windows were paper-thin single panes, and we could hear the traffic noise and people talking outside late into the night.

    We get up at 6:00 and have oatmeal for breakfast, then we need to buy groceries for my pre-race dinner, race day breakfast, and post-race meals. The grocery store is nearly a mile walk and we find most of the items we want—veggies, fruit, beans, and sweet potatoes. Also, we'd packed dry pasta from home along with my Ezekiel bread, peanut butter, honey, and banana for my pre-race breakfast.

    After returning to our Airbnb, we make lunch and then leave to research the subway system, so we will know how to buy tickets and which direction to travel to get downtown for the Race Expo. As we walk to the station, I realize my legs should be resting. With the walk to the grocery store and subway station, I decided to skip my 2-mile shake-out run today. Of course, with more than 30,000 runners and associated spectators heading to the Race Expo, the subway station is packed. There is also a delay due to an incident involving the police at the Alewife subway station.

    The subway system is easy to figure out with the information in English. It's not like traveling to another country and trying to figure out all the logistics in a foreign language. We arrive at the Race Expo and pick up my race bib. By that time my legs are getting super tired, so we catch a subway train ride back to our Airbnb to rest.

I meet three young women staying at our Airbnb who are also planning to run the Boston Marathon. Runners are assigned a wave and corral based on their qualifying race time. The young women are all in wave 3 which means they will need to be in their corral and start before me. I'm in wave 4 and my starting time is 11:00 so I'll get to sleep in and take my time getting to the marathon bus loading location in downtown Boston for my 8:45 bus. In the evening, Craig cooks up the pasta we brought from home, and, with the added veggies we bought, it makes a great pre-race-day fuel. As I try to doze off at night, my mind wanders all over the place and I have jittery feelings of anticipation for tomorrow's race. Finally, I sleep.

Countdown: 202 Days
Monday, April 15, 2019
<u>Boston, MA</u>

I woke up at 6:00 to the sound of thunder, the spectacle of lightning flashes, and a heavy downpour of rain.

I try not to be concerned. I've been tracking Boston weather for the last two weeks and I have been seeing a daily "no rain window of opportunity" and a bit of sun during my run time from 11:00 to 3:00. I eat my race day breakfast, a piece of toast with peanut butter, honey, and banana and I make a cup of coffee with hot water poured through a coffee-filled paper-towel "filter" into a cup. Our Airbnb has a coffee maker, but I couldn't find coffee filters, so I had to get creative. The coffee has a pretty weak taste, but it will be good enough for this morning.

I meet two of the other runners having breakfast in the common kitchen. We have a light conversation and end with "Good luck on your race," but we all seem preoccupied with the upcoming race. Craig is having his usual oatmeal and we still have plenty of time to get to the marathon bus which loads at 8:45. It's only a ten-minute walk to the subway stop and a 15-minute subway ride. It's 7:00 and I'm ready. Craig can tell I'm hyped up and jittery. He says we'll leave at 8:00 and still have plenty of time to get to the marathon bus. Rain is still pouring down as I put on my rain pants and rain jacket, and place my poncho and energy drink into my pack. I also pack a warm jacket, shirt, and dry socks for after the race. I give the pack to Craig. He suggests we take an Uber to the train station instead of walking and I feel much better with this decision to stay dry before the race.

As expected, it doesn't take much time to get to the subway station, downtown Boston, and the marathon bus loading location. Spectators aren't allowed on the bus, so Craig and I say our farewells in the loading zone. I give him kisses and a big hug as I leave him to make my way through security. Craig later told me that he felt a bit left out. He'd run the Boston Marathon three times, and this was the first time he'd been left behind as a spectator.

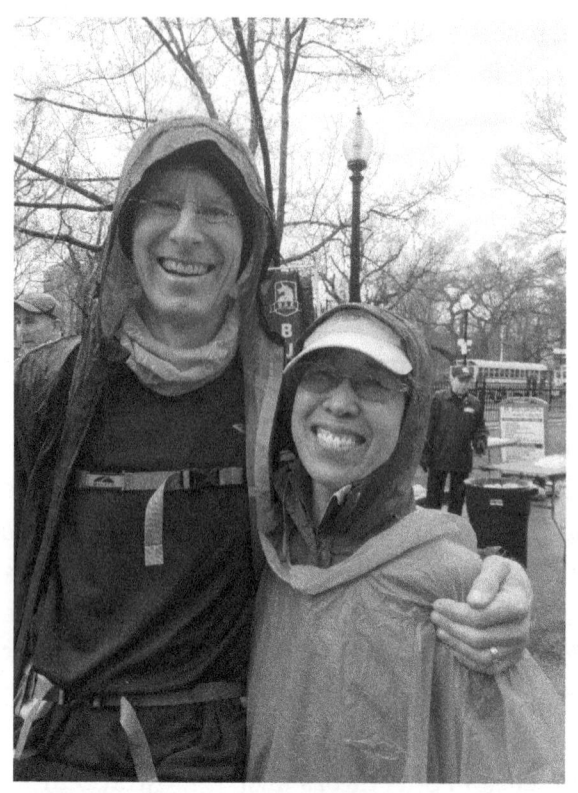

Before Getting on the Bus to Hopkinton

The bus ride takes over an hour to get to Hopkinton. When we arrive at the athletes' village there are thousands of runners and race officials, plus water and bagels for the runners. Luckily, the rain has stopped, however, many runners are wearing shoes covered with plastic since there's mud everywhere. I'm swept away with the other runners heading toward the race corrals. After the wave three runners start the race, it's time for the wave four runners to move into the corrals. Everyone is cheering and running toward the starting line. I see a few Koreans in my corral and say "Hanguk" (meaning Korea), give them a thumbs-up, and see smiles on their faces. The whole world is watching along with my family and friends who will follow my progress live on the Boston Athletic Association (BAA) mobile phone app. Boston is a magical place during this event and only a select few can stand where I'm standing right now.

When the gun goes off and I start running, I feel strong. The crowd of participants sweeps me along at a fast pace. Too fast? The raincoat I had tied around my waist and my gloves begin to feel too warm after a couple of miles. I take them both off and toss them on the side of the road. The first 15 miles seem easy. I hear the crowds cheering me (and all other runners) on. From mile 16 to 20, I'm tired but still doing okay. The weather that had been talked about so much leading up to race day ended up being perfect for running, with cloud cover and a temperature in the upper 60s. Miles 23 and 24 are a grind with my lower legs screaming. I feel like I'm barely moving. Then, suddenly, I have a comeback with more energy from mile 25 to the finish line.

How sweet it is to finish the Boston Marathon! I learned a few concepts of running:

- I could only faintly hear my coach in the back of my head telling me to go easy the first half of the marathon.
- It's too easy to start out too fast with the other fast moving runners sweeping me along.
- Late in the race, I need to focus on my mental strength rather than the pain in my legs.

I should be happy that I ran the Boston Marathon and happy for all the people cheering me on this journey, including my husband and coach, and my daughter Mira and son-in-law Pete, who drove down to Boston from Maine to see me after the finish. My granddaughter, Aria, son, Alex, and daughter-in-law, Nadya, cheered me on from their home in New York. They tracked my progress on their phone with the BAA app. However, despite the sweet feeling of crossing that finish line, it wasn't a stellar race for me. I finished with a time of 4:25 and a large positive split (i.e. the second half of the race took much longer than the first half of the race) at a 10:03 minute/mile overall pace. To be truthful, I feel disappointed by my finish time, which was much slower than my qualifying time of 4:11 at the Rome Marathon the previous year. I learned that I only have so much control over the outcome of a run. What I do know for sure is that I gave it my all leading up to race day with my training, my focus, and my dedication.

Countdown: 201 Days

Tuesday, April 16, 2019

Boston, MA

My legs are already feeling much better this morning. Not good enough to run another marathon yet, but better. Craig and I pack up from our Airbnb and take the subway into Boston for some sightseeing. It feels good to walk around a bit to help my recovery. Craig is hungry and we head to Whole Foods where we eat a morning snack. On the train and streets, marathoners are everywhere. They are easily identifiable by their 2019 light blue Boston Marathon jackets. I was an inconspicuous Boston Marathon runner since I did not purchase a jacket. After a bite of wholesome food, we go to Faneuil Hall Marketplace, Quincy Market, and Boston Harbor. We have a lazy afternoon and then head to Nancy and Jack's home in Concord, MA. Jack is Craig's second cousin once removed. We arrive around 5:30. Craig is put in charge of cooking dinner while the four of us talk about the marathon and life in general. Nancy and Jack's son-in-law was also in the marathon, but unfortunately, stopped early because of a pulled hamstring. One thing for sure about running 26.2 miles, you're running into "THE UNKNOWN." Anything can happen to anyone.

Countdown: 200 Days
Wednesday, April 17, 2019
Concord, MA

The weather is beautiful with a slight breeze. Jack is taking us on a walk to Henry David Thoreau's famous Walden Pond, only a few blocks from his house. I read "Walden" by Thoreau three years earlier and became influenced by his descriptions of his minimalist lifestyle, living on the northern shore of Walden Pond for two years, two months, and two days with only life's essentials. One of my favorite quotes from "Walden" is this one: "I went to the woods because I wished to live deliberately, to front only the essential facts of life, and see if I could not learn what it had to teach, and not, when I came to die, discover that I had not lived." I wonder how many people approaching death can truly say they have lived their lives fully.

Jack is a wealth of knowledge about both Walden Pond and Thoreau, and it is a great treat to hear him talk about them. It was a pleasant visit and a relaxing way to spend time after the race and before getting on the plane back to Colorado.

Countdown: 199 Days

Thursday, April 18, 2019

Colorado Springs, CO

Back at home, our refrigerator is empty. Craig is happiest when we're well stocked with food. Since I'm grounded from running for a couple more days, I help Craig with the grocery shopping. We make stops at Natural Grocers, Trader Joe's, and Costco. Loading up with vegetables, berries, fruits, and pasta brings a big smile to Craig's face.

Countdown: 198 Days

Friday, April 19, 2019

Colorado Springs, CO

I go to the gym for some much-needed stretching. I am recovering quickly from the marathon with no lingering discomfort. I'm not an elite, professional runner looking for financial gains. However, I love to run for my health, longevity, and the places running takes me. Also, running is my sanctuary time. I know that not everyone possesses the ability to run. I've been granted this gift and I want to make sure I use it.

Countdown: 197 Days

Saturday, April 20, 2019

Colorado Springs, CO

According to my coach, I'm finally able to run again today. "Easy and only four miles." It's a sunny, calm day and I enjoy my run without any training pressure. I don't remember when I last had this much fun running.

Countdown: 196 Days

Sunday, April 21, 2019

<u>Colorado Springs, CO</u>

This morning, I realize how much I have missed running on the trails in Ute Valley Park behind our house. It's wooded and quiet without the noise of traffic. Green leaves are opening up on tree branches and birds are chirping me onward. I'm running my favorite mid-mountain trail but have to watch out for the usual hazards of trail running—tree stumps, roots, and rocks. I pay attention to every step, every second. I almost trip twice but recover—yay.

Countdown: 195 Days

Monday, April 22, 2019

<u>Colorado Springs, CO</u>

Somehow my coach convinced me to run the Colorado Springs Triple Crown of Running race series. The Triple Crown consists of the Garden of the Gods 10-mile run on June 9th, the Summer Roundup Half Marathon in Cheyenne Mountain State Park on July 14th, and the Pikes Peak Ascent on August 24th. The Pikes Peak Ascent is 13.2 miles uphill with an elevation gain of 7,815 feet (2,382m). The race starts at 6,300 feet above sea level (1,920m) and finishes at the 14,115-foot (4,302m) summit of Pikes Peak.

I've run the Triple Crown of Running series before, in 2017 and 2018. I finished first in my age group both years. The 2018 Pikes Peak Ascent was disappointing because the race was cut short due to concerns over a potential afternoon thunderstorm. Race officials designated Barr Camp as the race finish line. My coach has convinced me to run it again as good training for the New York City

Marathon on November 3rd. My spring, summer, and fall are now all dedicated to my ongoing training.

Countdown: 194 Days

Tuesday, April 23, 2019

<u>Colorado Springs, CO</u>

 I run with the Pikes Peak Road Runner's Sunrise Striders this morning in Garden of the Gods Park. I'm up at 5:00, have my pre-run breakfast, and I'm out the door. Craig isn't running with me, so I drive there solo. I arrive at the main parking lot 10 minutes before the 6:00 start time. My fellow runners congratulate me on finishing the Boston Marathon. I hadn't realized so many local runners had watched the race.

 I see many familiar faces—Kevin, Ray, Jennifer, Mike, David, Josh, Stephanie, Darrell, and Ramsey. Many of them ask me where Craig is. I tell them he's cooking breakfast, haha. "You've trained him well," Kevin replies. To tell the truth, since Craig isn't training with me these days, he'll most likely eat seven pancakes and then go out for his leisure run in Ute Valley Park. I've never seen anyone eat so much before a run, but that's Craig.

 We start from the parking lot and do an easy run to Rampart Range Road (RRR). From there, we run hard 8-minute intervals up RRR followed by an easy downhill 4-minute recovery run and repeat this three times. We end up where we started at the base of RRR. I remember this tough training hill from before. I always feel so good after a hard workout, and I definitely get that feeling every time I run with the Sunrise Striders!

Countdown: 193 Days

Wednesday, April 24, 2019

Colorado Springs, CO

    I'm feeling cold and my nose is plugged up after yoga yesterday evening. The air conditioning was blowing right above my head during yoga practice. My body is not happy and is sending me a strong message. I make my special tea with homegrown sage, organic lemon, and local honey, drink it, and go right back to bed. I'm out for an hour and a half.

    I get up feeling completely recovered and go out to work in the garden. I empty the compost bin and spread the composted material into the garden, then turn over the soil to prepare for planting soon. Gardening gives me the same peace as running. There are other similarities, too. Gardening and running both require tons of care and training and they both provide me with bountiful rewards. You get back from life what you put into it.

Countdown: 192 Days

Thursday, April 25, 2019

Colorado Springs, CO

    I love my early morning training runs with the Sunrise Striders. Sometimes over 100 runners show up for these Tuesday and Thursday morning runs through Garden of the Gods. The runners divide into four groups, the fast Sunrise Striders, the middle pack, the trail social group, and the road social group. Today I run with the fast group over some technical trails. Because there are many elite runners, I'm nearly the slowest in the group. But since these are the elite runners, I feel it's okay even if I barely keep up. We warm up for four miles and then do 10x30-second intervals on a hill. I meet Maritz for the first time. She's a fast runner and I stay close to her the whole workout. She just returned from Germany and I learn that she's also signed up for the Triple Crown of Running series.

Countdown: 191 Days
Friday, April 26, 2019
<u>Colorado Springs, CO</u>

Another splendid day in Colorado Springs. When someone asks me where I want to live when I retire, I say, "Right here in Colorado Springs."

Countdown: 190 Days
Saturday, April 27, 2019
<u>Barr Camp Manitou Springs, CO</u>

I haven't been up to Barr Camp since December. It is a rustic bed and breakfast in the sense that you take your sleeping bag, sleep in a bunkhouse (outdoor lean-to or tent), use an outhouse, and skip showering. The year-round Barr Camp caretakers provide breakfast, and you can purchase dinner with your accommodations. I enjoy doing this but had stopped running up to Barr Camp to focus my training on the Boston Marathon.

This morning, I'm at Memorial Park in Manitou Springs at 5:55. Memorial Park to Barr Camp is a 4,000-foot vertical climb and the run is 14 miles round trip via the Manitou Incline. I already see a lot of runners heading toward the Incline, but I don't recognize any faces.

I run Lovers Lane through Manitou Springs to the bottom of the Incline. From there, I hike 39 minutes up the Incline at my regular pace. I'm glad to see I haven't lost any strength hiking up the Incline. I reach Barr Camp in a time of 2:09. Inside the cabin at Barr Camp, I see a friend and a familiar face, Jonathan, who congratulates me on my Boston Marathon run. Larry, who I just meet and who's hiking to the top of Pikes Peak, says he's buying me a cup of coffee to congratulate me on the marathon. I thank him and wish him a safe hike. I hear that there are copious amounts of snow on the trail above Barr Camp.

I eat my half sandwich (peanut butter, honey, and banana) and enjoy my free cup of coffee before I head back down Barr Trail to Memorial Park. On the trail, I run into Dave, who trains with Sunrise Striders. I give him a quick high five and clock my downhill run from Barr Camp to the train depot at 1:10. The train station is the home base for the cog rail train which has traveled up the mountain from Manitou Springs to the top of Pikes Peak (and back down, of course) for the past 125 years.

Countdown: 189 Days
Sunday, April 28, 2019
Colorado Springs, CO

As soon as I get up, I look for the London Marathon 2019 results. Eliud Kipchoge had an outstanding run and set a new London Marathon record with a time of 2:02:37. I admire his life philosophy, his focus, and discipline. I had no doubt he would win.

Today, Craig is presenting a workshop on "Why Food Matters," and my responsibility is to cook for 15 people. I do strength training in the morning at the gym, then cook up two main dishes, prepare desserts (oatmeal banana cookies and no-bake brownies), and cut up fruit. I am exhausted by the end of the day with barely enough energy to crawl into bed.

Countdown: 188 Days

Monday, April 29, 2019

<u>Colorado Springs, CO</u>

I run an easy five miles in Ute Valley Park this morning. The weather is cool and ideal, although I'm fortunate that I'm not one of those people who mind warmer weather. At home, I write and post a blog titled, "The Magic of Life and 26.2 Miles." <u>http://integratedlifestyletransformation.com/the-magic-of-life-and-26-2-miles/</u>.

Countdown: 187 Days

Tuesday, April 30, 2019

<u>Colorado Springs, CO</u>

I feel like I should steal Chinua Achebe's novel title "Things Fall Apart" for this entry. I run with the Sunrise Striders starting at 6:00 and when I reach the parking lot after my run, I'm the last one back and my car is the only one left.

The run went like this: It starts with light snow falling but about half an hour in, big fluffy snowflakes are completely covering my face and I can't see anything through my snow-covered glasses. I take my glasses off and can barely make out the runners way ahead of me. I remember today's training route—turn right on Pikes Peak Ave and continue for one and a half miles and then turn right onto Garden Drive to take me back to Garden of the Gods Park and the parking lot. I try to see the street signs and, at one point, I'm heading the wrong way. Thankfully, I'm familiar with the roads and I recognize Garden Drive and head up the hill. I run toward Balanced Rock where we're supposed to turn around and all the other runners have already made the turn. I'm at least ten minutes behind the last runner in my group. Perhaps I should be training with the "middle pack" runners. I could keep up with them. Since the Boston Marathon, I've been conducting a few experiments, such as running with faster runners to try and pace with them. I think I need to move back in the pack with runners who run at a similar pace. I feel terrible today and am not enjoying trying to keep up. Lesson learned, "know your limits."

Countdown: 186 Days
Wednesday, May 1, 2019
Colorado Springs, CO

A new experiment. In anticipation of a hard track workout tomorrow, I decided to take a total rest day without any running or strength training.

Countdown: 185 Days
Thursday, May 2, 2019
Colorado Springs, CO

It's cloudy and a cold 32°F at 5:00. I eat my usual pre-run toast with coffee and drive three miles to Garden of the Gods. Colorado Springs is such a playground for runners with all the different running clubs and trails. Today, I'm doing a nice, easy run with the Sunrise Strider's middle pack. I chat with Kathy and a new running friend, Sarah, who has three kids, aged four, three, and two. She's sure been busy during the last few years!

I enjoy this morning's run with the middle pack and think that, most likely, I'll stick with them. At home, I talk to Craig about my plan. He feels I should be with the fast Sunrise Striders. I'm going to have to go with my gut on this one, and it tells me the middle pack is the right group for me.

Countdown: 184 Days

Friday, May 3, 2019

<u>Barr Camp Manitou Springs, CO</u>

I'm up at 5:00, eat my pre-run toast with coffee, and head out the door for a long Barr Camp training run. I arrive at Memorial Park at 5:55 and run down Lover's Lane to the base of the Incline. It's perfect weather for this long run, a bit cool with no wind. I reach Barr Camp at 8:00 and meet two new Barr Camp caretakers, Mike, and Guillermo. Jonathan is there as well, painting the interior of the cabin before the overnight guests arrive in the afternoon.

I have a lovely conversation with Guillermo while eating my Barr Camp snack of half a peanut butter and banana sandwich and the best cup of coffee anywhere on the mountain (and the price is right at $1 per cup with free refills). On the way down, I notice the trail is quiet until I reach No Name, where I pass several spread-out walkers. I wiggle through them at a nice running pace and finish at the bottom feeling terrific.

Countdown: 183 Days
Saturday, May 4, 2019
Colorado Springs, CO

Today is a fun and exciting day for Craig and me. After strength training at the gym, we drive to Denver with our Toastmaster friend, Tom, to cheer on Greg, a Pikes Peak Toastmaster club member, and friend who is competing in the International Speech Contest at the District 26 Conference. Greg has already won the speech contest at the club, area, and division levels. During our drive to Denver, we have a lively conversation with Tom. At 24-years old, he is already a confident public speaker and is studying for his CPA exam. To top the day off, Greg wins first place at the conference.

I love competition at an individual level, where winning or losing is the responsibility of the individual and no other. No one can help you succeed or contribute to your failure. You rely entirely on yourself and how much you have poured your heart into the training. These principles apply to running as well as speech contests.

Countdown: 182 Days
Sunday, May 5, 2019
Colorado Springs, CO

I run on the trails in Ute Valley Park this morning. After a long drive and sitting in a conference room yesterday, I'm craving activity. New research finds that sitting is the new smoking, and I don't like to sit around for long periods. This morning's run shakes that inactivity out of my legs as well as the rest of me. It's pretty in the woods with a few mountain bikers riding the trails with me. They're all courteous, stepping off their bikes and moving to the side of the trail when I go by. It's a delight to share the trails with others.

Countdown: 181 Days
Monday, May 6, 2019

Colorado Springs, CO

    I help Craig with grocery shopping this morning. Normally, I don't drink coffee when shopping, however, I end up drinking a complimentary cup at Natural Grocers. It puts me on edge. These days, I can't handle even one cup of coffee without my head spinning. I used to drink several cups every day when I was in my corporate working life and it didn't rattle my nerves at all. Curbing my intake has decreased my tolerance.

Countdown: 180 Days
Tuesday, May 7, 2019

Colorado Springs, CO

    Rain is coming down softly, giving the ground some much-needed moisture. I can almost see the plants, trees, and grass smiling while drinking the raindrops. I love rain, even when I'm running. It always seems to cool me to an ideal running temperature. I'm in Garden of the Gods Park with the Sunrise Striders this morning. The temperature is in the 50s with light rain. The hilly terrain provides an excellent workout. In Colorado, we don't get many soggy days. The steady rainfall calms my mood and puts me in a tranquil space.

Countdown: 179 Days

Wednesday, May 8, 2019

Colorado Springs, CO

I cross-train today with 20 minutes each on the stationary bike, the elliptical machine, and the stair climber. This workout feels equal to my usual strength training and I hope I still believe this during tomorrow's run.

Countdown: 178 Days

Thursday, May 9, 2019

Colorado Springs, CO

Snow is coming down softly. It's cold and the trails are covered with fresh, wet snow. I'm running with the Sunrise Strider's middle pack and talking with Neira, who also ran the Boston Marathon. My shoes are heavy with mud, making each foot strike slippery. I have to stop and clean the mud off the bottom of my shoes the best I can on a rock and tree stump. I'm a bit lighter on my feet as we reach the asphalt road. Next, we run uphill, downhill, and uphill again. Everyone seems to pass me going uphill. I'm going to need to attack the ascents with more strength and speed.

Countdown: 177 Days

Friday, May 10, 2019

Colorado Springs, CO

I do a light workout at the gym and have a nice conversation with our good friend, Rod.

Countdown: 176 Days

Saturday, May 11, 2019

<u>Barr Trail in Manitou Springs, CO</u>

I do my long run up to Barr Camp early because Craig is presenting a workshop in the afternoon and I am the emcee. There are several inches of new snow and I'm the first person to break trail. I like to start early on my training runs—especially on long runs. I start today from Memorial Park at 5:30 and many runners are on their way up by the time I start down from Barr Camp around 8:30. I run into Maritz on my descent, talk with her for a few minutes, and I'm home by 9:50.

Craig's workshop is on "Mental Flexibility," an excellent topic, and I learn something new that I look forward to applying. It is a technique for suspending judgment by refusing to form a quick opinion or make an instant value judgment about something. Instead, one waits for more information or takes time to think the matter over, without the necessity of adopting a position about it immediately. Dr. Edward de Bono proposed a simple technique called "PIN." According to de Bono, one of the best ways to keep your value judgments under control is to respond to the new ideas and proposals of others in three distinct steps:

Step 1: Find something Positive to say about the idea.

Step 2: Find something Interesting about the idea.

Step 3: If you still feel the need, mention something Negative about the idea.

The advantage of the PIN formula is that it forces you to explore an idea in terms of its possibilities rather than its flaws. If you deliberately try to find something positive about the idea before you pass judgment on it, you run the risk of getting interested in it and may decide the idea has some merit after all. I'm going to make an effort to apply the PIN technique instead of reacting offhand to statements and possibly saying something offensive.

Countdown: 175 Days
Sunday, May 12, 2019
<u>Colorado Springs, CO</u>

I don't remember how long it's been since our neighbor, Randy, told us about the idea of planting the more temperature-sensitive garden plants on Mother's Day. I thought Mother's Day was a day for moms of all ages, to rest as their to-do list always seems endless, but Craig and I implemented the Mother's Day garden tradition anyway. We plant the tomato, pepper, basil, and cilantro plants. These store-purchased seedlings will provide an abundance of veggies and herbs during harvest and put smiles on our faces when we pick, taste, and nourish ourselves with them. It's so wonderful that nature provides us with everything we need if we're willing to work at it.

After planting, Craig takes me out on a date to the SunWater Spa in Manitou Springs. Craig and I watched the construction of the building for two years. We toured the establishment when they first opened, and today we're going to soak in several sun-heated, mineral-spring water tubs. We'll also enjoy a special, warm, saltwater bath. The Spa has a magnificent view of Pikes Peak and the Manitou Incline. It is a relaxing afternoon to follow the planting of the garden!

Countdown: 174 Days
Monday, May 13, 2019
<u>Colorado Springs, CO</u>

I am out at 5:24 for an easy 6-mile run. Because my schedule is full today, I'm getting my run in early. We all juggle our daily 24 hours, and my focus is running, rest, nutrition, work, and fun things like gardening and reading.

Countdown: 173 Days
Tuesday, May 14, 2019
<u>Colorado Springs, CO</u>

I am running in the Sunrise Striders middle pack at Garden of the Gods. It's nice running weather with no wind and a temperature in the upper 40s. The sun is about to rise above the horizon. I'm trying out my new Altra Superior 4 trail shoes. I love their light weight and how these shoes fit my feet. We start down Juniper Way Loop, and after warming up along Pikes Peak Ave, we run hill repeats on Ridge Road. Up, up, up, slow jog down, and up, up, up again. This is a long, gradual uphill and I'm out of breath each time at the top, but I feel great today and light on my feet in my new shoes.

I have a fantastic workout with Mike, Maritz, and Neira. I see Bernie, who has a swollen knee from last week's fall. Neira is complaining about her hip. We runners can be so addicted to our sport that even when our bodies send us clear messages about the need for rest, we ignore them and risk further damage. I tend to listen to my body's signals more carefully these days so that I can stay healthy and enjoy running. At the end of the day, if you're hurting you won't be able to fully enjoy the sport.

Countdown: 172 Days
Wednesday, May 15, 2019

Colorado Springs, CO

I'm finally having a cup of coffee with Michelle at The Perk Downtown. I met Michelle while competing in local races. She's really sweet. I hardly know her, except for our mutual encouragement to each other during races, but we've wanted to get together for a long time. She's just returned from travel with her parents in Peru and shows me her swollen Achilles tendon. She's been trying to take it easy on the running miles but is getting ready for the Wasatch 100 in early September. Yes, that really is a 100-mile race in the Wasatch Mountains of Utah with an elevation range from 4,400 feet to almost 10,000 feet. We discuss food, life, and running and make plans to run up to Barr Camp on Sunday, which I am excited about.

Countdown: 171 Days
Thursday, May 16, 2019

Colorado Springs, CO

I run with the Sunrise Striders this morning. Michelle encourages me to run with the fast group and I accept the challenge. We run hill repeats. I feel like it nearly kills me each time I get to the top, but it's a superb workout. Thanks, Michelle!

Countdown: 170 Days

Friday, May 17, 2019

<u>Colorado Springs, CO</u>

Things worked out well last time, so I'm cross-training at the gym again instead of my usual strength training. I bike for 20 minutes, work out on the stair climber for 10 minutes, and then do 10 minutes on the elliptical machine and finish the workout by stretching.

Countdown: 169 Days

Saturday, May 18, 2019

<u>Colorado Springs, CO</u>

Since I plan to run 4,000 vertical feet up to Barr Camp tomorrow with Michelle, I decide to run a relatively flat course today. I run down Centennial Boulevard to Garden of the Gods Road, down Sinton Trail, and back for a total of six easy miles.

Countdown: 168 Days

Sunday, May 19, 2019

<u>Barr Trail in Manitou Springs, CO</u>

It's colder today than it has been for the last few days with a temperature in the mid-30s. At 5:40 I run up Ruxton Ave alone and head up the Manitou Incline toward Barr Camp. Michelle, Robin, and I were planning to run up to Barr Camp together. Last night I got a text from Michelle saying she didn't feel well during a long run in Boulder, and had to check into an emergency room. Her fingers were tingling and she didn't feel right, so she had to cancel her planned Barr Camp run this morning.

I'd been excited to finally have an opportunity to train with Michelle and to meet her friend, Robin. Robin is in my age group, has been running fast, and beat me in the Winter Series Races by a large margin, but with Michelle's cancellation, I run solo today.

At the top of the Incline, I run into Steve, a daily Incliner. He recently won his age group climbing up the stairs in the Empire State Building Run-Up Race. This is a famous race up the 1,576 steps (86 flights). I congratulate him and continue my run to Barr Camp. My time to Barr Camp is 2:06, my fastest time this year. I was able to cut off three minutes going up and four minutes on the way down with a 1:06 descent. My strength and speed are improving. My Barr Camp goal by the time I run the Pikes Peak Ascent on August 16 is 2:00 up and 1:00 down.

Countdown: 167 Days

Monday, May 20, 2019

Colorado Springs, CO

I feel great after yesterday's 14-mile run up to Barr Camp (and down), despite the vertical elevation gain of 4,000 feet. Today I'm cross-training—bike, stair climber, and stretching. It looks like winter is back with freezing rain, snow, and wind. Before I leave for the gym, I cover my precious and delicate herbs. Craig came up with a creative idea to cover the peach tree by pinning an old shower curtain around it. He used old sheets to cover the strawberry plants. Living in the Rockies, you can expect all types of weather regardless of the season. What I know for sure is that the "season" is nothing but a suggestion for the weather.

Countdown: 166 Days

Tuesday, May 21, 2019

<u>Colorado Springs, CO</u>

Winter is back. We got dumped on with six inches of wet, sloppy snow overnight and my training schedule this morning calls for a tempo run with the Sunrise Striders in Garden of the Gods Park. I wake up at 4:45, see snow-covered streets and snow still coming down hard, and go back to bed. Craig asks me what's up. I tell him about the weather, and he volunteers to drive me if I'm worried that the road conditions are too treacherous. I decide to go for a run near home, knowing that the tempo run isn't a good idea for today's conditions.

I run down the street in deep, wet, sloppy snow and find that with every footstep water and snow are splashing all over my shoes and ankles. The wind suddenly picks up and blows into my face. I regret not wearing my face mask this morning. I run in the car tracks on the road, pushing snow out of the way with each step, mindful to watch for approaching cars. As soon as I see one, I move to the edge of the road to avoid the splatter from the car as it passes. Spring training for sure.

Countdown: 165 Days

Wednesday, May 22, 2019

Colorado Springs, CO

We're traveling to Ossining, New York (one hour by train north of New York City) to visit our granddaughter, Aria, and of course, my son, Alex, and daughter-in-law, Nadya. We're up at 4:00 to drive to the airport and today will be a rest day for my faithful body.

Countdown: 164 Days

Thursday, May 23, 2019

Ossining, NY

I love the Ossining High School track and every time I visit, the gate to the track is open. I haven't done a track workout since training for the Boston Marathon, so this is a good training opportunity. I run 6x800 meters followed by a 2-mile cooldown. Compared to the 6,500-foot altitude of our home in Colorado Springs, the less than 200-foot elevation in Ossining makes a big difference, and the 40 and 50°F weather in New York is a very nice change from the cold, wintry weather in Colorado Springs.

Countdown: 163 Days

Friday, May 24, 2019

Ossining, NY

Today is a rest day and we are out shopping for tomorrow's party. My daughter-in-law has such a loving family. They get together often and celebrate with good food. Nadya, Aria, and I are grocery shopping while Craig stays behind to work on the installation of their newly-delivered dishwasher. After removing the 30-year-old dishwasher, there are plenty of surprises. The house was built in the 1930s, and the delivery personnel can't install the new dishwasher with the old copper pipe and old wiring. Craig is great at solving challenging problems and coming up with creative solutions, a quality that I admire in him. The delivery team leaves and, one trip to the hardware store later, Craig finishes the installation.

Countdown: 162 Days

Saturday, May 25, 2019

<u>Ossining, NY</u>

 I'd planned to run 10 miles today, but it's pouring rain. I didn't see rain in the forecast before I packed for our New York trip and didn't bring a raincoat. I wait a few minutes and the rain begins to clear up, almost stopping.

 I'm familiar with the quiet route, surrounded by big trees. On Farm Road, I see wild turkeys. Everything is so lush, with the entire world wrapped in my favorite shade of green. I run up Long Hill Road East, a steep hill. Hills are my best friends when I'm training. Next, I tackle Long Hill Road West. It's turned out to be a good hill-training run today.

Countdown: 161 Days

Sunday, May 26, 2019

<u>Ossining, NY</u>

 I am up at 5:45 and out for an easy run. It's early with few cars, which makes running at this time of day enjoyable. Flowers are in full bloom: rhododendron, lilac, iris, and azalea. It's like heaven on earth, and bike riders encourage me as they pass saying, "You're moving pretty well." Many people have a false, preconceived notion of New Yorkers being rude. I see the kindest New Yorkers during my runs. In general, people are good and kind regardless of location.

Countdown: 160 Days
Monday, May 27, 2019
<u>Ossining, NY</u>

I have been totally in the moment spending time with our 22-month-old granddaughter, Aria. We have only a few more hours to spend with her before we get on the train. She is amazing to observe. She absorbs every word I speak and every movement I make. Together, we do all the yoga poses I can think of. Aria loves doing yoga. She is a natural, requiring little effort to do child pose, three-legged dog, sphinx, and tree poses. I wonder how a baby can so easily embrace all the information. Is her brain that uncluttered and ready to record everything that is happening in her environment? At last, the time comes to end our visit with family and fly back to Colorado.

Countdown: 159 Days
Tuesday, May 28, 2019
<u>Colorado Springs, CO</u>

I am in Garden of the Gods at 6:00 with the Sunrise Striders and looking forward to our run. They push me to my maximum whenever I run with them. Also, it's really fun to see all the familiar faces, find out what is happening in the running world with my friends, and catch a glimpse of their lives. It's an energetic, enthusiastic group.

Countdown: 158 Days
Wednesday, May 29, 2019
Colorado Springs, CO

It is an easy cross-training day at the gym.

Countdown: 157 Days
Thursday, May 30, 2019
Colorado Springs, CO

Today's run with the Sunrise Striders is a warmup followed by 25 minutes of hard running up Rampart Range Road. The road isn't too muddy today, except for a few wet spots from yesterday's thunderstorm. I am last up the road with the fast runners and still climbing while they are already coming down. The descent requires fast leg turnover, and since the Boston Marathon, my leg turnover on the downhills is getting much better.

Countdown: 156 Days
Friday, May 31, 2019
Colorado Springs, CO

Today is an easy gym day.

Countdown: 155 Days

Saturday, June 1, 2019

<u>Golden, CO</u>

Craig and I have arrived at the Colorado School of Mines Steinhauser Fieldhouse in Golden, CO for the REVEL Rockies Expo. I pick up my bib and race packet for the half marathon tomorrow. We watch a presentation by a REVEL coach. He gives a few pointers and goes over the course for both the marathon and the half marathon. The course is all downhill, with a 4,708-foot drop in altitude for the full marathon and a 1,693-foot drop for the half marathon. I absorb two important tips from coach Paul.

1. For the entire race, stay at effort level 7 on a scale of 1 to 10, with 10 being maximum effort.
2. Run the "tangents." That is, minimize the race distance by aiming for and running the inside corner of every turn. There are many turns on this winding mountain road.

We are grateful that Denver residents, Kayla (Craig's daughter), and her boyfriend, Robert, join us for dinner at Chipotle. A cardinal rule for running a race is to not change anything from the regular training routine, especially food, drink, racing clothes, shoes, and fuel. I have never eaten at Chipotle before any running race, so I am following the cardinal rule. I have brought my pasta from home and eat it as my pre-race day dinner.

Countdown: 154 Days

Sunday, June 2, 2019

<u>Evergreen, CO to Morrison, CO</u>

I have the run of my life today with a half marathon finish time of 1:47:32:10 at an 8:12 minute/mile pace!

Craig and I get up at 4:00 and I eat my usual pre-run piece of toast with peanut butter, honey, and banana with a cup of coffee. I pack my coffee from home (cardinal rule) but can't find a coffee maker in our Airbnb. I improvise by pouring my pre-ground coffee and water into a cup. I heat it in the microwave for a minute, let it sit for a few minutes, and filter the coffee through a paper towel into a second cup.

We drive to the parking lot in Morrison designated for racers and spectators, where I load onto a bus for the ride to the starting line in Evergreen. I kiss Craig as I get on the bus at 4:45. He will be waiting for me at the finish line after his 5-mile run in Morrison and after eating the six pancakes he packed for himself. The bus ride from Morrison to Evergreen is a different experience than the pre-Boston Marathon bus ride. During the Boston ride, the runners' energy was through the roof and I could hardly hear myself think. However, this ride from Morrison to Evergreen is so quiet it seems as though no one is awake. I arrive in Evergreen with all the runners shouldering their Expo pre-race foil blankets. We are one hour away from the start time.

I line up in the long bathroom line. The wait is good because it helps the time go by. Next, I line up behind the starting line under the 1:50 finish time sign. I chat with Jennifer, who calls me "Boston" since I am wearing my 201 Boston Marathon shirt. Jennifer tells me she is tryin' qualify for the 2020 Boston Marathon. As we run together Jennifer encourages me by saying, "Let's go Boston!" The race is all downhill and I soak up the beautiful, wooded mountain scenery and peaceful sounds from Bear Creek, which follows the road and the course. I run the Revel Rockies half marathon as a long-distance training run and set a personal record for the half marathon distance (1:47:32), breaking my previous record by nearly 12 minutes.

Countdown: 153 Days

Monday, June 3, 2019

Colorado Springs, CO

I'm amazed to feel so good after my hard run yesterday. My body needs a rest, and I am off to the gym for some light cross-training with the stationary bike, stair master, and stretching.

Countdown: 152 Days

Tuesday, June 4, 2019

Colorado Springs, CO

This week is the final week of training with the Sunrise Striders in Garden of the Gods before the 10 Mile Garden of the Gods race. I see Michelle and she introduces me to Tracy, another ultra-distance trail runner. We do a 4-mile warmup on the trail followed by 10x30 second hill repeats. The fast runners have already finished their 10 hills when I have finished eight. We run less than half of a mile around the inside Garden Loop and repeat the hills. I complete my two sets of hill repeats. Michelle comes over for breakfast after the run. It's fun to chat with her about running and her nutrition. I make her five servings of "superfood for runners" prepared with love—sweet potatoes, beets, beans, onions, garlic, and turmeric. It's a fun morning and I am grateful to connect with Michelle.

Countdown: 151 Days
Wednesday, June 5, 2019
<u>Colorado Springs, CO</u>

The day has escaped me. It has now become a good rest day.

Countdown: 150 Days
Thursday, June 6, 2019
<u>Colorado Springs, CO</u>

It's a fabulous day. Craig has decided to join me in running with the Sunrise Striders. It's the last training day in Garden of the Gods. I love the "Garden" training runs. The park is only a five-minute drive from the house and the scenery is amazing when the sun pokes through the red rocks. We run only 3.5 miles and finish with coffee and snacks.

Countdown: 149 Days
Friday, June 7, 2019
<u>Colorado Springs, CO</u>

Craig and I go to the Colorado Running Company store to pick up my bib for the Garden of the Gods 10-Mile Run on Sunday. Craig's goal this year has been to run no races and just give his body a rest. We wait in a brief line at the back of the store before I am handed my bib. Craig remains at the front of the line as if he is expecting something. A moment later, he is handed a bib. I don't understand at first, but then I'm surprised and thrilled that Craig is running the race "with" me. It's much more exciting to go to an event when I know Craig and I will be participating together.

Countdown: 148 Days
Saturday, June 8, 2019
<u>Colorado Springs, CO</u>

Another magnificent day and rest day in the "Springs."

Countdown: 147 Days
Sunday, June 9, 2019
<u>Colorado Springs, CO</u>

The Garden of the Gods 10 Mile Race starts this morning at 7:00. The weather is a bit chilly with the temperature in the low 40s and wind gusts up to 15 mph. I have on a long sleeve shirt and windbreaker, gloves, and a winter hat. This is a terrific race and convenient with the start/finish line and parking only three miles from our home. The race is only 10 miles and provides amazing views of the park. I run my heart out and come in 2nd place in my age group. But when I see my time, I realize I haven't improved my time in this race over the last three years (2017 - 9:09 minute/mile pace, 2018 - 9:11 minutes/mile, 2019 - 9:12 minutes/mile). I've been training so hard, and I'm sliding backward. I feel like I'm failing. Is this normal? It makes me want to question everything. What is this running all about? If I keep failing, why do I still keep running? What can I do? Do I need a new coach?

Countdown: 146 Days
Monday, June 10, 2019
Colorado Springs, CO

Today is gym day and an easy rest day as I recover from yesterday's race.

Countdown: 145 Days
Tuesday, June 11, 2019
Colorado Springs, CO

My morning is consumed with meetings, so I run in Ute Valley Park at lunchtime. The heat has risen to 76°F. I run in shorts and a short-sleeve shirt for the first time this year. It is great to feel the heat after the cold, snowy, wintery spring-training runs. With the heat and time of day, I feel sure to run into rattlesnakes. Snakes are not my friends, especially on the trails. When I come across one, my tactic is to yell "snake" to scare them away. If that fails, I try to jump over them. Luckily, I am not treated to any snake encounters today.

Countdown: 144 Days
Wednesday, June 12, 2019
Colorado Springs, CO

Strength training at the gym.

Countdown: 143 Days

Thursday, June 13, 2019

<u>Manitou Springs, CO</u>

Craig and I are meeting our running friend, Rod, at 7:00 at Memorial Park in Manitou Springs for a run up to Barr Camp. We are 20 minutes early, as usual. My motto is "If you can't be on time, be early." With Rod's health issues I am in the lead at the Incline and up to Barr Camp. About four minutes after I reach Barr Camp, Rod and Craig show up. Whoever reaches Barr Camp first buys coffee for everyone else. This is the first time this year I have had the privilege of buying coffee!

Countdown: 142 Days

Friday, June 14, 2019

<u>Frisco, CO</u>

Craig and I are heading to Leadville, CO (elevation 10,151 feet) to see Craig's daughter, Kayla, race in the Leadville Heavy Half—so named as it's a 15-plus-mile race instead of the usual 13.1-mile half marathon. This year, the officials have changed the course due to too much snow on the trail at the higher elevations. Yes, Colorado did have a very cold and snowy winter.

This will be the first time in Leadville for us since Craig attempted to run the Leadville Trail 100 Run in 2012, back when we were dating. I was supposed to pace Craig after midnight at both the Outward Bound and May Queen aid stations, but he got behind the cutoff time at Twin Lakes aid station after 67 miles and 20 hours and did not complete the race. We're not racing this time, though. We're just going to enjoy running local trails there.

When we arrive in Frisco to eat dinner at Whole Foods, I get a text from Kayla and her boyfriend, Robert, saying they are having car trouble. They happen to be in Frisco, only two blocks from us. So, we box up our food and meet them at a pizza restaurant. Robert's sister, Gina, is running the race with Kayla and all three of them are stranded. We give Kayla and Gina a ride to Leadville so they can get to the race-packet pickup before it closes for the evening. Robert remains in Frisco until his dad arrives and changes cars with him, then rendezvouses with us in Leadville. Robert's dad is able to slowly drive Gina's car with a failed turbocharger back to Denver. I'm grateful that Craig and I were there to help out Kayla and Gina. The universe always seems to be putting us exactly where and when we need to be. It is damp and rainy as we drive back to our Silverthorne Airbnb.

Countdown: 141 Days

Saturday, June 15, 2019

Leadville, CO

The weather has improved from last night and is a perfect 50°F for race day. Craig and I queue up at the starting line with Kayla and Gina. We will run with them for a portion of the race. Craig plans to run three miles out and three back. I plan to run five miles out and five back. The course starts with a significant climb and Kayla and Gina have already started walking. Craig slows down to stay with them. I run ahead. I see so many runners from Colorado Springs. I can't believe I know so many runners everywhere I go.

The course is a gravel road and dirt trails with rocks. The scenery is beautiful. I turn around at five miles and wait for Kayla and Gina. I decide to start running back and some runners think I am the lead runner. I don't feel good about running the course without a bib. I should have signed up for the race and run the whole course, but it was a fun day. Robert, a mountain biker, did a 40+ mile training ride at high elevation with thousands of feet of vertical climb and descent. Kayla and Gina both finished the race with smiles on their faces.

Countdown: 140 Days
Sunday, June 16, 2019
Colorado Springs, CO

I run six miles from our house on a hilly out-and-back trail. The long uphill trail follows Flying W Ranch Road up over Mountain Shadows Pass and then down the other side. I turn around and run up and over Mountain Shadows Pass a second time. It is sunny and warm. I hope this is the beginning of some pleasant spring weather. I enjoy running in shorts and short sleeves.

Countdown: 139 Days
Monday, June 17, 2019
Colorado Springs, CO

Today is a total body rest day. No running and no gym.

Countdown: 138 Days

Tuesday, June 18, 2019

Colorado Springs, CO

    The weather is finally warm enough to ditch the winter hat and gloves. I do a tempo run this morning—one easy warmup mile, then 20 minutes of running at my 10k race pace and finishing up with a 1-mile cooldown. My body feels good today.

    Later, I have a cup of tea with Alisa, Rod's wife, to see how they're both doing. I've been concerned about Rod's health since Thursday's Barr Camp run when he struggled going up the Incline. I am once again reminded that without health, you lose everything.

Countdown: 137 Days

Wednesday, June 19, 2019

Colorado Springs, CO

    Today is a total rest day in preparation for tomorrow's long run. I've been trying out a different routine by doing a total rest day rather than going to the gym before a long run.

Countdown: 136 Days

Thursday, June 20, 2019

Bottomless Pit Sign on Barr Trail Manitou Springs, CO

    Craig and I run up to the Bottomless Pit sign on Barr Trail, about one mile above Barr Camp. I believe this will be great training for our upcoming Cheyenne Mountain State Park Half Marathon and the Pikes Peak Ascent, the second and third legs of the Triple Crown of Running race series. I feel refreshed and think my total rest yesterday helps my performance today. I shave one minute off last week's run to Barr Camp for a time of 2:05.

Countdown: 135 Days

Friday, June 21, 2019

Colorado Springs, CO

I do my regular strength training at the gym today with plenty of stretching.

Countdown: 134 Days

Saturday, June 22, 2019

Colorado Springs, CO

Running in Ute Valley Park is always peaceful. I don't have to listen to traffic noise or maneuver through traffic lights; I just keep watch to make sure I don't run into wild animals. All I see today are a few deer and one mountain biker. The trail is in perfect condition thanks to just the right amount of rain lately—enough to control the dust, but not enough to create mud puddles. My mind wanders and I enjoy the many purple wildflowers and lush green grass. It seems my 6.3-mile run is over quickly this morning.

A guest from NY is staying at our Airbnb and has decided to climb Pikes Peak. Craig provides him with five pancakes, two no-bake brownies, and fruit, and loans him gloves and a water bottle. He starts his ascent at the trailhead at 4:00 a.m. and we don't see him again until 6:00 p.m. He tells us it took him 10 hours to reach the summit, hiking through wind gusts and blowing snow near the top. When he returns to the house, he is nearly hypothermic. He stays in the shower for over 30 minutes until the hot water runs out, but he is so happy he accomplished his goal despite the weather and his lack of conditioning. And we were happy to see him return safely with his goal accomplished.

Countdown: 133 Days
Sunday, June 23, 2019
Colorado Springs, CO

The temperature is cool, in the low 40s, and there is a breeze. I feel like I could run forever this morning. After last night's rain, I smell the fragrance of the Russian olive trees lining a portion of the trail. I decide to run by Wilson Park and up to the Blodgett Peak trailhead. The road is quiet with few cars. I planned to run eight miles and I end up running 8.67 miles, feeling great.

Countdown: 132 Days

Monday, June 24, 2019

Colorado Springs, CO

It is a strength training day at the gym.

Countdown: 131 Days

Tuesday, June 25, 2019

Colorado Springs, CO

It is sunny, in the 50s with no wind, and ideal weather for interval training on the trail near our house. So different from my January Boston Marathon training days! The trail is dust-free, ice-free, and snow-free—perfect. My half-mile interval times in January on the icy, snowy, windy trail were in the 4:30s. My times today are all in the 4:10s. I'm happy with my progress but would like to cut another 10 seconds off my times before the New York City Marathon. I need to do more research on improving speed.

Countdown: 130 Days
Wednesday, June 26, 2019
Colorado Springs, CO

My goals for running are health, traveling with a purpose, seeing places I wouldn't otherwise have thought to go, and connecting with nature. I prefer trail running over road running, being alone, and running in a peaceful place where I can be in tune with my breathing and footsteps. Today is all that.

Countdown: 129 Days
Thursday, June 27, 2019
Colorado Springs, CO

I start my run at 5:00 enjoying the 70°F weather. Again, I am running without gloves. I am so happy to be running in light running gear compared to my heavy winter running clothing.

I run down Sinton Trail for the first time since the Boston Marathon. The snow is gone, and the trail is lined with verdant vegetation. I feel the tall grass against my hands and brush the grass seeds at the top of the shoots. I see a couple of bikers and one runner.

Countdown: 128 Days
Friday, June 28, 2019
<u>Colorado Springs, CO</u>

Today is a light day at the gym with stretching in anticipation of tomorrow's long run. I've already started thinking about my Saturday run with Michelle. We are planning a trail run up to the A-frame on Pikes Peak. The A-frame is a shelter at tree line (12,098 feet, 3,687m elevation), three-quarters of the way up Barr Trail, and three miles from the summit of Pikes Peak. It's ten miles from Memorial Park in Manitou Springs to the A-frame and the run will be part of my Pikes Peak Ascent training.

Countdown: 127 Days
Saturday, June 29, 2019
<u>A-Frame on Barr Trail, Manitou Springs, CO</u>

Rod and I are at Memorial Park at 4:50 with plans to meet Michelle and friends at 5:00 for our training run to the A-frame. We chat while watching the time. It's 5:01. Rod and I look around the parking lot and don't see Michelle. I tell Rod, it's time to go. I don't wait for anybody. The corollary to "If you can't be on time, be early," is "If you are late, you better be fast enough to catch up." I don't expect anyone to wait for me, especially when they are starting a long run. I run with Rod for only a mile before he takes off, leaving me behind. I can only imagine how fast he was in his prime.

Just before No-Name (four miles up), Rod is coming down the trail looking deeply disappointed. He tells me he got a call from work and must check in at 7:00. I ask him to look out for Michelle and her friends, describing Michelle as looking Asian and shorter than me. He's surprised to hear that anyone is shorter than me!

I continue to Barr Camp in a time of 2:16 and arrive at the A-frame at a modest time of 3:16. This is my first longer run up Barr Trail and I'm happy with the time. On the way down, I run into John and Joe. Wow, so many people I know on the trail today. Finally, at a half-mile above Barr Camp I hear Michelle's voice, "Is that you, Hae?" Yay. I hand her the homemade power bar I prepared for her and continue down. I take a break at Barr Camp for hot tea and my half sandwich. It's getting warm and busy at Barr Camp as I leave. I maneuver around the train of hikers as I run down the trail. The busy trail indicates summer is in full swing.

Countdown: 126 Days
Sunday, June 30, 2019
Colorado Springs, CO

My legs feel good after yesterday's long run. At the gym I focus on strength training, stretching, and giving my legs a well-deserved rest.

Countdown: 125 Days
Monday, July 1, 2019
Manitou Springs Incline, CO

My 16 weeks of New York City Marathon training officially started today. I'm up at 5:00 and have my pre-run breakfast with coffee, grab my CamelBak with 16 ounces of water, and am out the door. Instead of doing a tempo run today, I decided to train on the Incline.

I need to be alone for my hard workout as today is the 10th anniversary of losing my first husband to a heart attack. It was one of the darkest moments in my life and it seemed at the time there was nothing I could do to ease my sorrow and heartbreak. After Chris's passing, I found running as a way to cope with my pain. I started running the trail behind my house in Park City, UT, often with tear-filled eyes, unable to see the trail or where I was going. Bit by bit, time and running started to heal my wound.

I met Craig in late 2011. He had already done his share of running and I was just beginning my journey. We shared our joy of running together and set a goal to run a marathon together on all seven continents. That goal has taken us to so many magical places—South Africa, Patagonia (Chili), New Zealand, and Rome. I'm grateful that running has been part of my journey of healing, both mentally and physically.

Countdown: 124 Days

Tuesday, July 2, 2019

<u>Colorado Springs, CO</u>

I am off to the gym today for strength training and afterward will pack for our mini-vacation to Rocky Mountain National Park and the surrounding area.

Countdown: 123 Days

Wednesday, July 3, 2019

<u>Kremmling, CO</u>

After driving to Kremmling, we stay overnight in an economical Airbnb. We're up early this morning to run before we continue our drive through Grand Lake, Rocky

Mountain National Park, Estes Park, and Loveland on our way to our next overnight stop in Fort Collins. Kremmling offers many dirt trails for jeeps and ATVs, but the roads are empty early this morning and completely belong to Craig and me. Craig is reminded of Immigration Trail in Park City, UT, a wide gravel road with rolling hills. I agree. It's a peaceful run this morning, followed by a spectacular drive through a tree-covered mountainous landscape. We make several stops to view and take pictures of the scenery, and to walk in Grand Lake and Estes Park.

Countdown: 122 Days
Thursday, July 4, 2019
Fort Collins, CO

I love water—the oceans, rivers, and streams. Water calms me and helps me achieve a peaceful mind. Craig and I have the opportunity to run from our Airbnb this morning through the neighborhood to a 21-mile paved and single-track trail along the Cache la Poudre River (French: hide the powder). The name comes from the 1820s when French trappers hid their gunpowder along the banks of the river during a raging blizzard.

The river is flowing full and fast from all the snow that fell during the winter. My mind wraps around the gentle sound of the river and I feel as though I could run forever on this trail. Craig turns around at two miles, but I continue for a bit. I try to catch up with another runner on the trail. Yes, I pass her as my watch shows three miles, and I turn back. Amazingly, I don't get lost in the neighborhood on my way back to the Airbnb. Quite an accomplishment for me.

Today we drive west and north of Rocky Mountain National Park through the Never Summer Mountain range. The Never Summer Mountains have a breathtaking view, and I'm not sure why they aren't a part of Rocky Mountain National Park. We stay at an Airbnb in Hayden, CO, a reasonably priced and very clean hostel that's only 30 minutes from Steamboat Springs.

Countdown: 121 Days

Friday, July 5, 2019

<u>Steamboat Springs, CO</u>

Craig and I plan to run up to the top of Werner Mountain this morning. The weather is perfect with plenty of sun, no wind, and temperatures in the low 60s. Steamboat Springs is a magical place that brings back all the memories of my 50-mile Run Rabbit Run Race, the first race I ever signed up for. I think we are running up the same trail that we ran up in 2013. When I finished the Run Rabbit Run Race tears were flowing down my face at my sense of accomplishment and the human capacity for resilience. Today, I am in a different frame of mind, with no race and no stress. I have been running more miles than ever and I have grown more confident as a runner.

Compared to our September 2013 Run Rabbit Run Race, the warm summer season brings us more and larger green vegetation. I see many perfect fiddleheads along the trail, which I pick for dinner this evening. Fiddleheads are immature fern fronds about to unroll for the season. I wish my oldest sister, Mung Son, were here with me. She would be in heaven. She's a medicine woman who knows all about nature and wild edible plants.

I think I have picked enough for dinner. I stop and, while waiting for Craig to catch up with me, put them in my CamelBak pocket. We eat them for dinner with beans and quinoa and they're delicious.

Countdown: 120 Days

Saturday, July 6, 2019

Hayden, CO

We head home from our Steamboat Springs vacation. Craig and I listen to 26 Marathons, an audiobook, by Meb Keflezighi and Scott Douglas. There are great lessons from the professional marathoner in this book on setting specific goals for a given race and never giving up, even when you hit the wall. Meb won both the Boston and New York City Marathons during his career and I admire his determination.

Countdown: 119 Days

Sunday, July 7, 2019

Colorado Springs, CO

Our mini-vacation is over and we're home. I'm running Flying W Ranch Road for the good hill-climb training and loving it. While driving home, we also listened to ChiRunning: A Revolutionary Approach to Effortless, Injury-Free Running by Danny Dreyer. Danny provided great tips on running with flow, not with resistance. So today I try to run with a relaxed and proper posture to help me feel light and run with less effort.

Countdown: 118 Days

Monday, July 8, 2019

Colorado Springs, CO

I enjoy easy strength training at the gym today.

Countdown: 117 Days

Tuesday, July 9, 2019

Colorado Springs, CO

Another gorgeous day for hill repeats with sunny skies, no wind, and 54°F at 5:45. I warm up with a slow jog one mile north to the Ute Valley Park sign and back, then I run up the hill into the park, beginning my 8x hill repeats. There are several people on the hill this morning. Almost halfway through, two men show up running alongside me. I am a bit faster than the two guys. "You're killing it," one says. I have seen both of them working out at Accolade Gym. It's always nice to encounter familiar faces on the trail.

Countdown: 116 Days

Wednesday, July 10, 2019

Colorado Springs, CO

After my Toastmasters meeting I am much later to the gym than usual. It's crowded and noisy when I get there, and I am anxious to finish my routine and leave this congested space. It's not that I'm antisocial, but I prefer the gym quieter and less busy.

Countdown: 115 Days

Thursday, July 11, 2019

<u>Colorado Springs, CO</u>

I'm up at 4:30 this morning for my scheduled 10-mile run. I've decided to run to the Garden of the Gods from our home. I haven't been there since the Garden of the Gods 10 Mile Race in June. The Garden always provides me with the right diversity of training, combining hills, both up and down, with asphalt roads and gravel trails. I easily run through the variety of terrain and manage to bring the perfect amount of water for today's run, 8 ounces.

Countdown: 114 Days

Friday, July 12, 2019

<u>Colorado Springs, CO</u>

We have two boys, five and three years of age, and their dad visiting us from Evergreen, CO. I have to say, I'm exhausted from watching the kids this morning. They're full of energy and require constant attention. I don't remember this much work watching my kids at their age.

After our guests leave, my stress dissipates at the gym when I do my strength training. It was fun, though, to see the kids' unspoiled innocence and pureness. I feel like running puts me in the same state of innocence and purity. When I run, I'm not concerned about anyone's thoughts about me, or my thoughts about anyone else. It's just me, alone.

Countdown: 113 Days

Saturday, July 13, 2019

<u>Colorado Springs, CO</u>

I do a 3-mile shakeout run this morning in preparation for tomorrow's half-marathon race in Cheyenne Mountain State Park. I leave my Garmin watch behind as I don't want any disturbances from Strava notifying me of other athletes' workouts. I need to focus on tomorrow's race and quiet my mind with no distractions. I'm not even sweating after three miles and I feel great. I get home just in time for Craig's famous, blueberry-oatmeal pancakes with berry compote—my favorite breakfast after running.

Countdown: 112 Days

Sunday, July 14, 2019

<u>Cheyenne Mountain State Park—Colorado Springs, CO</u>

Today is the Summer Roundup, the second leg of the Triple Crown of Running race series. The Summer Roundup is a half marathon up and down the side of Cheyenne Mountain State Park on single-track trails. Since the weather gets warm quickly in the morning, race officials are starting the race at 6:30 rather than the previous year's start time of 7:00. The course is rugged, with a fair amount of elevation gain (and loss), rocks, and tree roots.

Craig is running with me today and we see many familiar faces at the starting line: Rod, Verena and John, Ray, and Bernie. Race officials allow runners to line up according to their anticipated minute/mile race pace, starting with an 8-minute/mile pace, to alleviate the bottleneck at the beginning of the trail. We start in the asphalt parking lot and run uphill on the road before turning onto the single-track dirt trail. I start the race with Rod who lines up behind the 9-minute/mile sign. Rod is still a fast runner and in his prime, he ran a 2:20 marathon. Unfortunately, lining up according to our anticipated pace didn't do enough to mitigate the congestion when we turned onto the single-track trail. Perhaps the race officials will come up with a new idea next year. My goals are to:

1. Set a new course record for my age group.
2. Be first place in my age group.

The sun is already beating down on us when the race starts. The heat and hills take a toll on me. Despite that, I achieve my two goals and am happy with the results. Craig also did better than last year but he is laying down after the race and complaining about leg cramps. I give him water, watermelon, and oranges along with a light massage on both legs.

Countdown: 111 Days
Monday, July 15, 2019
Colorado Springs, CO

I feel so good. It's as if I didn't even run yesterday. I believe I am getting stronger every day. It is gym day today with strength training and stretching.

Countdown: 110 Days

Tuesday, July 16, 2019

<u>Manitou Springs, CO</u>

I train with the Sunrise Striders on Barr Trail today. We're doing 4x8 minutes of hard uphill running with a 4-minute easy uphill jog in between intervals. I am surprised to see so many runners show up at 5:45, including my friend Michelle. Michelle introduces me to her friend, Josh, whom I had heard of but not met. We start at Memorial Park with a 1-mile warmup run up Ruxton Avenue. I am behind the elite runners. Michelle and Josh are behind me. Michelle is tapering for her Never Summer 100k race in two weeks, so she is not pushing herself. I've fallen behind everyone by the time I get to No Name (4.3 miles) and turn around, but it's still good training.

Countdown: 109 Days

Wednesday, July 17, 2019

<u>Colorado Springs, CO</u>

I am coaching my friend, Lili, who ran her first 5k race last month. She was so excited about placing 5th in her age group in her first race. She called and asked me if I would train with her on the hill into Ute Valley Park, the hill she will be racing up next Friday in her second race. I spend time with Lili on the hill. She ran her first 5k in 36:31 on the hilly, single-track trail. We set a goal for her to cut her time down to 35:00 minutes for the second race.

Countdown: 108 Days

Thursday, July 18, 2019

<u>Bottomless Pit Sign—Barr Trail, Manitou Springs, CO</u>

Spoiler alert, I didn't make it up to the A-frame today. The heat wasn't my issue. It was much cooler high up on Barr Trail than the nearly 100°F in Colorado Springs. Still, my Incline and Barr Camp times were slow, and my body didn't want to move today, especially my legs. I realize I made a big mistake training Lili yesterday evening. Normally, I go to the gym and rest on Wednesdays. Lesson learned. Don't alter the training schedule.

I make it up to the Bottomless Pit sign (seven miles up Barr Trail), and come down to Barr Camp, where I wait for Craig. Craig planned to run up to the A-frame, three miles from the summit. I ask a few hikers and runners to deliver the message to Craig if they see him on the trail that I'm waiting at Barr Camp. Finally, Craig shows up, smiling. I can tell from his expression that he had a great workout. Coming down, I have a decent 7-mile run. The heat feels scorching as I descend into Manitou Springs, but I don't mind. I remember how much I shivered during my winter and spring training runs.

Countdown: 107 Days

Friday, July 19, 2019

<u>Colorado Springs, CO</u>

The heat is still on and I go to the gym for my stretching and strength training. I run into Dave, one of the leaders of the Sunrise Striders running group. He seems to be on the phone the whole time he is at the gym. I don't know what it is about all of us with our devices and technology.

We can't seem to get away from them for even an hour. How about disconnecting from the "technology/device/business" while we work out?

I love escaping from all my daily activities when I run or do strength training, giving me total "me" time with nature or the gym equipment. It is truly a precious gift of time for my mind and body, and I love it. I am grateful for technology and we live in an extraordinary time. On the other hand, all human inventions have pros and cons. I'm sure we'll look back on this time 50 years from now and see how the Internet has both helped and harmed the human race.

Countdown: 106 Days

Saturday, July 20, 2019

<u>*Manitou Springs High School Track, CO*</u>

Today is my first day on the track since the Boston Marathon. The temperature is already 72°F at 4:30 but, again, I would rather have the heat than the ice and cold. I will run a 1-mile warmup followed by 4x400m, with a recovery run of 200m between each interval, 2x800m with a recovery run of 400m between each interval, 4x400m, with a recovery run of 200m between each interval, and then run a 1-mile cooldown. My fastest time today for 400m is 2:00 minutes, a couple of seconds behind my interval pace in March. I think I can pick up the pace. I have experimented with Danny Dreyer's ChiRunning technique, focusing on form, arm movement, core strength, and breathing. I like his philosophy of running injury-free and working with Chi (energy). A couple of my running friends have injuries and continue to run. It is so hard to stop, even with pain or discomfort. For me, I will continue to work on the techniques of ChiRunning.

Countdown: 105 Days

Sunday, July 21, 2019

Colorado Springs, CO

I run six easy miles today. It seems my speed is not improving since the Boston Marathon. I need to rethink and strategize my speed training. My goal is a sub-9 minute/mile marathon pace, and my pace today is around 9:45 minutes/mile.

Countdown: 104 Days

Monday, July 22, 2019

Colorado Springs, CO

Today is stretching and strength training at the gym.

Countdown: 103 Days

Tuesday, July 23, 2019

Colorado Springs, CO

Early morning, nice and cool, is the best time for training runs, especially hill repeats. My hill repeats are quick and hard and then I cool down by running a few miles. I run into Steve and Lu, our neighbors, taking an early walk in Ute Valley Park.

Countdown: 101 Days
Thursday, July 25, 2019
<u>Colorado Springs, CO</u>

I am out at 5:15 this morning. It's dark and I use a headlamp. I run long today, starting with three miles along 30th Street to Garden of the Gods Park. Although early, I see a lot of runners and a large group of walking soldiers. Colorado Springs is home to the Air Force Academy, Fort Carson, and Peterson Air Force Base. I carry just the right amount of water for my 12-mile run, 16 ounces. When I get home, Craig is in his regular clothes and greets me from the kitchen as I enter the house. He has already finished his run and is cooking his oatmeal-blueberry pancakes and cutting up fruit to go with them. When I finish my shower, breakfast is ready and being served. I am a lucky girl. We both sit out on the front porch, eating pancakes and fruit. We have a beautiful morning as Craig takes a stroll through memory lane telling me about his fast time in the Women's Nike Marathon in California and the Ocala Marathon in Florida.

Countdown: 100 Days
Friday, July 26, 2019
<u>Colorado Springs, CO</u>

In preparation for tomorrow's Pikes Peak Ascent training, I work out at the gym and make my running fuel, which consists of coffee blended with dates, peanut butter, and honey. I also pack a peanut butter, banana, and honey sandwich for after the run and three homemade power balls made out of oats, maple syrup, cacao, and bananas. I'm usually anxious the day before a big training run, but today I feel relaxed. I'm breathing easy and planning to have a good night's rest.

Countdown: 99 Days

Saturday, July 27, 2019

Pikes Peak 14,115', CO

We reach the summit of Pikes Peak at 10:20. We'd planned to start our run at Memorial Park in Manitou Springs at 5:30 but begin, instead, at 5:40. Rod is fiddling with his water bottles and his car key, then tells us that he is going only halfway up to the summit, making his turnaround point, Barr Camp. He said he was not ready for the summit today.

Craig is waiting for me at Barr Camp and asks if I want to continue. I do. The 2.6 miles and 2,000-foot elevation gain from Barr Camp to the A-frame can be a real grind due to the thin air, rocks, and tree roots, but I keep up with Craig today.

I keep telling myself, that if this is hard for me, then it's hard for others too. The trail does not have any favorite person. I drink plenty of water along with my fuel. At the A-frame, I suggest to Craig that we take a quick break and a little of our food. We stop for just 30 seconds. I eat one power ball which gives me the energy to continue up. The next three miles are even more difficult. I run into Justin, a friend from the Sunrise Striders group. He is hiking with someone slower, so I pass both of them. After 4 hours and 47 minutes (4 hours and 38 minutes for Craig), we reach the summit. It was a slow day to the top, but we accomplished our goal. At the end of the day, that's all that matters. We hitchhike down the road and find a ride within 30 seconds of putting our thumbs up. A nice young couple from Georgia and Missouri give us a ride into Manitou Springs where our car is parked. I am so grateful for the kind people in this universe.

Countdown: 97 Days
Monday, July 29, 2019
Colorado Springs, CO

I leave the house at 5:30. It is 60°F and just right for running in shorts and a short-sleeve shirt. I need to take advantage of the good weather, knowing that the cold mornings will soon be here. I run one easy warmup mile up Flying W Ranch Road. This mile has a 180-foot elevation gain, a grind, but I feel good. The workout today is a breeze compared to Saturday's Pikes Peak summit. I'm happy with my run this morning.

Countdown: 96 Days
Tuesday, July 30, 2019
Colorado Springs, CO

It is a travel day to New York to celebrate our granddaughter's second birthday. We get up at 4:00 and drive to Denver International Airport to catch a flight to LaGuardia Airport.

Countdown: 95 Days

Wednesday, July 31, 2019

Ossining, NY

    We are in Ossining, New York, an hour train ride north of Manhattan. The weather is hot and muggy. However, I must continue my training. The days are getting shorter and the countdown to the New York City Marathon is now in the double digits. The time is going by so fast!

Countdown: 94 Days

Thursday, August 1, 2019

Ossining, NY

    We are in Ossining with another hot and muggy day for training.

Countdown: 93 Days

Friday, August 2, 2019

Ossining, NY

    Today is a rest day. Craig and I go to Aria's school with her parents to celebrate her second birthday. The 10 two-year-old kids are fun to watch. Their language and speaking skills are hard to understand, but their expressions are priceless.

Countdown: 92 Days

Saturday, August 3, 2019

Ossining, NY

    I run 13.2 miles starting at 5:15. It rained last night, and everything is still wet, including the roads. My clothes are soaked due to the humidity and air temperature in the 70s. Traffic is light this early on a Saturday morning, giving me a break from constantly looking out for cars.

Countdown: 91 Days
Sunday, August 4, 2019
<u>Ossining, NY</u>

Today is a rest day in Ossining.

Countdown: 90 Days
Monday, August 5, 2019
<u>Ossining, NY</u>

I'm thrilled to be back on the Ossining High School track. I run 400m intervals and set a PR at 1:55 minutes, probably helped by the extra oxygen at sea level.

Countdown: 89 Days
Tuesday, August 6, 2019
<u>Colorado Springs, CO</u>

After returning from New York, I crave trail running. I run in Ute Valley Park, enjoying nature, peace, quiet, and fresh air.

Countdown: 87 Days
Thursday, August 8, 2019
<u>Manitou Springs, CO</u>

Craig and I are meeting Mikko at Memorial Park in Manitou Springs at 6:00 for our Incline to No Name training run. I am up at 5:00, have a quick cup of coffee, and a piece of toast, and am ready to head out. Craig, on the other hand, is cooking and taking time to eat six pancakes and a pile of fruit for breakfast. While he is eating, he's watching a video at the breakfast table, knowing he has plenty of time. I am a solo trainer and don't like working around others' schedules. I love the freedom of getting up and heading out.

We are 15 minutes early getting to Memorial Park and I decide to go for a slow 1-mile jog while Craig waits for Mikko. He shows up on time and we jog to the base of the Incline. I PR on my Incline ascent in a time of 37:31 and continue to up No Name. While I wait at No Name, halfway to Barr Camp, our friend, John, comes down from Experimental Forest. When Mikko and Craig show up, we run down Barr Trail to end a fun training morning.

Countdown: 86 Days
Friday, August 9, 2019
Colorado Springs, CO

It's a gorgeous morning and I begin to sense fall just around the corner. The temperature feels cool, although it's in the 60s. I have not been to the gym for a week as we were in New York for our granddaughter's birthday.

Countdown: 85 Days
Saturday, August 10, 2019
Colorado Springs, CO

Craig and I plan a 3-2-1 training run from the top of Pikes Peak. The training involves a 3-mile run from the summit down Barr Trail to the A-frame, a run back up to the summit, a run down two miles, and a run two miles back up to the top, then a 1-mile run down, and a 1-mile run back up. I hope the weather will hold off until we finish. We frequently have thunderstorms in the afternoons in Colorado Springs and even earlier in the day at the summit of Pikes Peak. I pack a rain jacket in preparation for the weather.

We arrive at the Pikes Peak Highway toll gate at 6:40. A few cars are already in line ready to go through. A volunteer tells us the gate will not open until 9:00 for visitors to the top of Pikes Peak because of a bike race. We decide not to wait around and drive part way home to Red Rock Canyon Open Space. It has been a year since we ran here and there are many nice trails with plenty of uphill and downhill variety. We run six miles and return home. We'll try the 3-2-1 workout again tomorrow.

Countdown: 84 Days
Sunday, August 11, 2019
<u>Pikes Peak 14,115', CO</u>

We fail again on our second attempt at the 3-2-1 workout, this time due to the weather. We start at Pikes Peak summit at 8:22 feeling good, running downhill with fresh, morning energy. After last night's rain, in the first mile down there are waterfalls and small streams across the trail as it switches back and forth. The rocky trail is slick as I jump over the puddles of water. We run down to the A-frame (three miles) and run back up to the summit. I wish I could have this much energy during race day. I would run my fastest time. Even though we're running between 12,098 feet and 14,115 feet, I feel fresh running uphill for only three miles.

I've just turned around, starting '2' of the 3-2-1, when Craig meets me near the top and says that the weather is moving in. We return to the summit and go into the visitors' center to regroup. The concern about the weather is twofold. One, lightning can be deadly and two, blowing rain and dropping temperatures can induce hypothermia.

Ray comes into the visitors' center while we are sitting at a table. He started his run from Manitou Springs. He's still breathing rapidly and is out of energy. We decide to run down to the Devil's Playground (12,780 feet) parking lot at road mile 16 where our car is parked. We hike the first part of the trail down from the top, which is all boulders and slippery rocks and not well defined. As we pass about one mile, the trail becomes runnable to the parking lot. I see many runners doing a 3-2-1 training today. Many of the participants in this year's Peak weekend (Pikes Peak Ascent/Marathon two weeks from today) have the same idea we did.

Countdown: 83 Days

Monday, August 12, 2019

Colorado Springs, CO

It's good to be back in the gym and doing some strength training. I read an article about a 71-year-old Korean woman setting the world record for the half marathon in a sub 1:40 time. I hope I can be as fast as her before I am 70 years old! The idea of being 70 sounds scary but maybe not if I can reach it in the same shape she's in. Wow, I'd better not waste any time.

Countdown: 82 Days

Tuesday, August 13, 2019

Colorado Springs, CO

    I am doing 8x hill repeats up Steep Mother this morning. Other runners show up with the same idea. It's less than two weeks until the Pikes Peak Ascent (Saturday) and Marathon (Sunday), and many participants are here today and training hard. I run an easy 2-mile warmup and solid hill repeats. Although I don't set any PRs on the uphill, I feel strong today. I end with another 2-mile cooldown. Craig and I do a one-hour yoga practice in the evening to finish up a productive training day.

Countdown: 81 Days

Wednesday, August 14, 2019

Colorado Springs, CO

    I skip the Toastmasters meeting this morning. If I sit in a meeting for more than an hour, the sun will be beating down and it will be hot for a run. I love to run early in the morning in the pre-dawn darkness. I can barely make out objects in the street and it's usually nice and cool. I run two miles and the sun begins to rise and everything becomes visible. I practice ChiRunning today, focusing on breathing and form. As my mind wanders, I refocus. I run 8.45 miles at a 9:46 minute/mile pace. This is acceptable. I am building endurance with this run, not speed. I'll need both for the Pikes Peak Ascent race on August 24th.

Countdown: 80 Days

Thursday, August 15, 2019

<u>Pikes Peak 14,115', CO</u>

This is our last training run from the summit of Pikes Peak before next week's race. The sunny weather is cooperating this morning with no clouds in sight. A large herd of bighorn sheep, ewes, and lambs, greet us as soon as we reach the top of the mountain in the shuttle bus from the Devil's Playground parking lot. Wow, what a treat it is to see these beautiful animals.

We're planning on running down three miles to the A-frame and back up to the top. It's an easy workout and I'm relaxed and confident. On the downhill, I fly through the boulders. Running back up, though, requires different muscles and strength. Craig looks strong today and passes me near the cirque at 13,300 feet. We both train well today.

Countdown: 79 Days

Friday, August 16, 2019

<u>Colorado Springs, CO</u>

I'm in taper mode (reduced quantity of running) before the race and go to the gym for a light strength-training workout.

Countdown: 78 Days

Saturday, August 17, 2019

<u>Colorado Springs, CO</u>

I run Ute Valley Park this morning. Everything is cool and fresh after yesterday's afternoon shower. The wild sunflowers are in full bloom this time of the year reminding me that fall is around the corner, and that summer will be ending soon. There are a lot of mountain bikers riding on the trails this morning. I step off the trail and yield to the bikers when they come by even though the bikers are supposed to yield to runners. It is easier for me to step off the trail, rather than for bikers to stop and restart.

Countdown: 77 Days

Sunday, August 18, 2019

<u>Colorado Springs, CO</u>

I am entering maximum taper mode. The coach is allowing only two days of running this week and only three miles on each of those two days. Taking a break from running and getting into a relaxed mode for a week will be a difficult challenge for me.

Countdown: 76 Days

Monday, August 19, 2019

<u>Colorado Springs, CO</u>

In addition to tapering for the Pikes Peak Ascent, I'll be focusing on healthful nutrition, good sleep, and rest this week. The temperature today is in the 60s and the weather is welcoming for running. I run four miles on the neighborhood trail this morning as three miles just wasn't doable for me.

I see Dave on the trail, running much faster than I am. If you start young (Dave is in his 30s) and train hard, you will continue to be a fast runner later in life.

Countdown: 75 Days

Tuesday, August 20, 2019

Colorado Springs, CO

It is an undemanding strength training day at the gym.

Countdown: 74 Days

Wednesday, August 21, 2019

Colorado Springs, CO

I am out at 4:45 with a headlamp. It's dark, windy, and warm at 61°F. I have a Toastmaster's meeting at 6:44, so I decide to run early. The trails are quiet, and it is only nature and me. I run up to Centennial Boulevard where the streetlights illuminate the sidewalk and road. I run four miles again, even though my coach told me to run no more than three. The warm breeze brushes my face and hands. I feel alert and refreshed running in the dark. I have a couple of early dog walkers for company. Dogs are great that way. They not only give unconditional love but can also get their owners out for an early morning walk.

Countdown: 73 Days

Thursday, August 22, 2019

Colorado Springs, CO

I am resting today and eating tons of organic beets, which grow big and healthy all summer long in our garden. Craig is adding some chopped greens to his pancake mix. I regularly add beets to my dishes and, today, mix beet greens and beets to our brown rice and lentil pasta for lunch and dinner. I love the sweet flavor of beets and the bitter taste of beet greens. We have learned that the nitrates in beets reduce oxygen expenditure during exercise. Therefore, this week is perfect for incorporating lots of beets into our diet with the upcoming race. Every little bit adds up to better results.

Countdown: 72 Days

Friday, August 23, 2019

<u>Manitou Springs, CO</u>

We pick up our race packets for tomorrow's Pikes Peak Ascent. There is a festive atmosphere in Manitou Springs with runners and vendors inside the Expo tent. Since the Pikes Peak Marathon, on Sunday, is one of Salomon's Golden Trail Series races this year, it has drawn elite runners from all over the world and I'm getting excited about the race. This will be my second Pikes Peak Ascent. In 2017, I finished second place in my age group with a time of 4:24:15. I ran again in 2018, but the race was shortened to finish at Barr Camp, so this will only be my second time running the full Ascent. Also, I've been training hard for the New York City Marathon and this race is part of my training.

I see Michelle at the Expo. She plans to run the Pikes Peak Marathon (up and down Pikes Peak) on Sunday. It's good to see she is all smiles. Her goal is to finish first in her age group. My goals are as follows:

1. Top three in my age group.
2. PR with a time of 4:20:00 or better.

I prepare my usual power drink along with a couple of items that will meet me at the top—a down coat and food. The forecast looks good for the race and I am ready to go.

Countdown: 71 Days

Saturday, August 24, 2019

<u>Pikes Peak 14,115', CO</u>

Wow, I blew it. I didn't meet either of my two Pikes Peak Ascent goals. I came in fourth place in my age group with a time of 4:38. I am not sure what went wrong. I need to seriously reassess my training (core, strength, cross-training, running), nutrition during the race, taper, and mental preparation.

Going into the Ascent I thought I had trained well, but perhaps not optimally. Our last and most critical 3-2-1 training run was cut short because of the potential for severe weather. I did complete rests Thursday and Friday for my taper. The energy drink I used during my long training runs (8 ounces of coffee, honey, dates, and peanut butter) was too sweet this time and my body rejected it. Also, I had to stop for 45 seconds to pee, something I never had to do during my training runs. I was almost dizzy after the A-frame and couldn't think straight. Perhaps it was the high altitude and maximum exertion of race day, but I had been training at high altitude without this issue. The wind was blowing 35 mph, but that's not unexpected. Nevertheless, I could hear Rod's voice in my head saying, "Keep moving" which was his tip of the day before the start of the race.

I saw many familiar faces before the start. Jen and Mike came out to cheer the runners, and Rebecca and Steve were cheering the runners from their driveway on Ruxton Avenue. Rod, Ray, Susan, and Tracy were all at No Name, Lori at Bob's Road, and Ling, Teresa, Jonathon, and Reagan at Barr Camp. I felt fortunate to know so many volunteers and spectators. When I finally reached the summit, I was surprised to see Craig sitting on a rock at the finish line waiting for me. Our plan was for the first one up to wait for a minute or so and get on a shuttle to meet the other person at Glen Cove (road mile 13) where we would catch a bus ride together to Manitou Springs. Craig was feeling unwell from the exertion and altitude, so we quickly boarded a shuttle to head down. He said his left knee was going numb and he could neither eat nor drink anything.

When we got down to Glen Cove, a bus was waiting for us to take us the rest of the way down to Manitou Springs. Of course, my sweetheart, Craig, wanted to sit next to me, so we asked another runner if he could move to another seat. When we arrived in Manitou Springs, families and friends of runners were all waiting and watching the finish line on the big screen. Patty was handing out finisher's shirts when we went into the Expo tent to pick up ours. Since her retirement, she looks beautifully happy. By now Craig was able to drink some water, lay on the grass beside the food tent, and stretch. We ran into another resting runner and gave him our beer and food tickets. At least we made him happy with all the extra tickets.

I am glad we finished the Triple Crown of Running Series with podium positions for both Craig and me—first in my age group for the series and third for Craig in his age group. The big lesson from today's race is to reassess my training and nutrition for the New York City Marathon, now less only 71 days away.

Countdown: 70 Days

Sunday, August 25, 2019

Manitou Springs, CO

It is a fun rest day for us as we go to Manitou Springs to watch the Pikes Peak Marathon runners finish their race. I hope Kilian Jornet from Spain will set a new course record. We hear he is 2:09 at the summit and expect him to be down around 10:30. He comes in at 3:26:58 with the fifth-best Pikes Peak Marathon finish time. The record marathon time, 3:16:39, was set by Matt Carpenter in 1993. We watch Sage Canaday cross the finish line in second place with a time of 3:39:09. It is amazing to watch Maude Mathys crush the women's course record. She finishes at 4:02:41 breaking Megan Kimmel's 2018 marathon course record of 4:15:06 by nearly 13 minutes. These top finishers are competing in Salomon's Golden Trail Series. It's so fun cheering all the elite runners as they cross the finish line that I nearly lose my voice from all the yelling.

Countdown: 69 Days

Monday, August 26, 2019

Colorado Springs, CO

I start hill repeats at 5:45. It is dark with the sunrise coming at 6:20. A warm wind blows into my face and I am still not happy about my weekend race results. I decided to look at my training schedule to see where I might tweak it. Also, I choked on nutrition starting at tree line (the A-frame). My body was rejecting the energy drink. It was way too sweet and not going down. I had an empty stomach and no energy to climb the rest of the way to the summit. Lesson learned regarding energy drinks for race day.

Countdown: 68 Days

Tuesday, August 27, 2019

Colorado Springs, CO

I do a tempo run. My legs feel a bit tired still, so I cut the training short and look at tweaking my core strength training. There are many approaches to core strength training, and I want to pick an effective technique for running. I am looking at the single-leg deadlift, single-leg bridge, lateral lunge, and side planks.

Countdown: 67 Days

Wednesday, August 28, 2019

Colorado Springs, CO

Another total rest day with research on core strength training. I find some good exercises, again with the single-leg deadlift, bridge, and abdominal workouts. I have been missing all these core workouts. It's never too late to incorporate exercises that might enhance my running, so I'll add three or four of these workouts into my routine.

Countdown: 66 Days

Thursday, August 29, 2019

Colorado Springs, CO

I am back to training on the roads for the New York City Marathon. I run from our house to Garden of the Gods Park starting at 5:45. The sun will be poking above the horizon about the time I get to the Garden. As you know by now, I love early morning runs. It's so quiet, the air is fresh, and there are no distractions. It is just nature and me.

When I get to the Garden, I find the trail closed because of a large flood water mitigation project. Sometimes when a trail is closed I can get through, but this one is closed off with a wire fence. I turn back and continue running into the park on the road. From Gateway Road onward, I feel much better not competing for road space with cars. I make a loop around Balanced Rock before heading home.

Today, I try something new for my energy fuel. Craig picked up a few Spring Energy gels yesterday from the Colorado Running Company store. I drink one gel down with water at mile seven and continue to feel good. My body is not rejecting the gel and I have good energy for the next seven miles. The morning is cool with ideal running weather. I feel great after my 14-mile run today and still feel energized when I reach home.

Countdown: 65 Days
Friday, August 30, 2019
Colorado Springs, CO

A complete rest day today.

Countdown: 64 Days
Saturday, August 31, 2019
Colorado Springs, CO

I go out for an interval speed workout; 10x half-mile intervals with a slow half-mile recovery in between intervals. My half-mile interval time seems okay, with an average of 4:13. Craig says my average half-mile interval time means I'll run 4:13 in New York. Hmmm... that does not seem so speedy anymore.

Countdown: 63 Days

Sunday, September 1, 2019

San Francisco, CA

    Craig and I fly to California to celebrate our fifth wedding anniversary. We plan to spend time in Yosemite National Park, Mammoth Lakes, South Lake Tahoe, and Berkeley. I get up early to run an optional (according to the Coach's schedule) six miles. It's dark out and I don't want to carry a headlamp, so I run along Centennial Boulevard and Garden of the Gods Road where both roads are lit with streetlights. This is a new route for me. When I get home, I take a quick shower and enjoy the pancakes Craig made for me. Food is so delicious after working out.

    We leave for the Denver airport three hours before our direct flight to San Francisco. At the San Francisco airport, we rent a car and drive to our Airbnb in Sonora. On our drive through the farmland of central California to Sonora, we see many fruit and veggie stands along the road. The almond trees lining the road are loaded with nuts. This is a first for us to see almonds on trees. We stop and purchase the freshest, most delicious peaches and figs, along with almonds fresh off the tree. What a treat to enjoy fresh fruits and nuts. I am in heaven.

Countdown: 62 Days

Monday, September 2, 2019

Yosemite National Park, CA

    Craig and I are excited to see El Capitan and Half Dome in Yosemite National Park this morning. We get up at 4:00, eat oatmeal and fruit for breakfast, and arrive at Yosemite National Park around 6:00. No one is at the park entrance gate and we already have a lifetime pass, so we drive right in. California is famous for traffic at toll booth entrances to national parks and we feel fortunate to avoid waiting in line. We decide to run a few miles in Yosemite Valley. We run to Mirror Lake and back. It is an amazing day with spectacular park scenery.

Countdown: 61 Days

Tuesday, September 3, 2019

<u>Mammoth Lakes, CA</u>

    I have read about fast and famous runners training in Mammoth Lakes where the elevation of nearly 7,900 feet gives the runners an advantage. These runners include Denna Kastor, who won the women's bronze marathon medal at the 2004 Olympics in Athens, Greece, and Meb Keflezighi who won a silver marathon medal at the 2004 Olympics, won the 2009 New York City Marathon, and won the 2014 Boston Marathon, becoming the first American man to win both the New York City Marathon and the Boston Marathon since 1983. I know that Tim Tollefson, a fast, ultra-distance runner, runs on the same Lake Mary Road I'm running on today. At 7881 feet, Mammoth Lakes is a bit higher than our home in Colorado Springs, which sits at 6,500 feet. Mammoth Lakes is known for high winds, but today is unusually calm. Craig and I run up to Twin Lakes, a running destination our Airbnb host recommended. It's so beautiful here and we enjoy the good conditions for a great morning run.

Countdown: 60 Days

Wednesday, September 4, 2019

<u>South Lake Tahoe, CA</u>

Lake Tahoe is beautiful and South Lake Tahoe is bustling with tourists. Even though Labor Day weekend, a couple of days ago, is the unofficial last weekend of summer, summer hasn't yet ended here. We cross the California/Nevada state line and rent a little cottage for two nights for our anniversary. South Lake Tahoe has an organic grocery store called Grass Roots Natural Foods where we buy organic fruits and veggies. Craig is thrilled to find an organic grocery store, knowing that we can buy and consume delicious fruit and vegetables without compromising the nutritional value of the produce with pesticides and chemicals.

We drive to Emerald Bay, a beautiful and popular spot for photography. We hike up to Eagle Lake, a round trip of two miles. After lunch, we drive to the Lake Aloha Trailhead of the Pacific Crest Trail at Lower Echo Lake. We do a short 4-mile run, but Coach warns me that it's my rest day today. Wow, we ran on the Pacific Crest Trail, even if for only two miles out and back. I feel darn proud.

Countdown: 59 Days

Thursday, September 5, 2019

<u>South Lake Tahoe, CA</u>

Coach has me out for an 18-mile long run today. Yesterday, he and I scoped out the trails long enough for today's run and we found the perfect running/biking trail along Lake Tahoe Boulevard.

Craig drops me off at Pioneer Trailhead at 5:50. It's dark with another half hour before sunrise. I plan to follow the trail along Lake Tahoe Boulevard and then turn onto the trail along Emerald Bay Road. At nine miles out, I will turn around. The bike trail is well-lit with streetlights. After running four miles, the trail disappears and I am lost. I find a way out to Emerald Bay Road and the adjacent trail and continue running on the trail until the time to turn around. When I am three miles from completing my run the coach drives by and says, "Hi babe," as he heads to the Pioneer Trailhead to pick me up. What great timing. When I am at mile 18, I find Craig walking toward me. I finish my long run, ready to stop but feeling strong and like I didn't expend any great effort at a 10:01 minute/mile pace.

Countdown: 58 Days
Friday, September 6, 2019
<u>Berkeley, CA</u>

On our way back to the San Francisco airport, we spend a night at an Airbnb in El Sobrante, near Berkeley, where Craig had many work trips. He shows me the Skates on the Bay restaurant where he and his work associates would dine the night before they spent a long day working at the Lawrence Berkeley National Laboratory. It must have been fun for him to see his old haunts.

I see some great running trails by the bay. I also see many people camped out, and homeless. I feel sad seeing the trash along the bay near the camps, but then again, picking up trash might be the last item on the campers' priority list. Likely, they do not have a priority list and are just living in the moment and taking care of the essentials, such as feeding a hungry stomach or finding shade to avoid the scorching hot sun... Life's priorities are different for every single one of us.

Countdown: 57 Days
Saturday, September 7, 2019
Colorado Springs, CO

It is wonderful to travel, and yet, it is comforting to be home with clean air and quiet trails. I do half-mile intervals today.

Countdown: 56 Days
Sunday, September 8, 2019
Colorado Springs, CO

Today is a total rest day from running. Craig and I go to Garden of the Gods Park and hike the Siamese Twins trail.

Countdown: 55 Days
Monday, September 9, 2019
Colorado Springs, CO

I run 10x hill repeats early this morning at the entrance to Ute Valley Park. It's dark, but I can make out the trail without a headlamp. I think about encountering black bears, as they live here in the nature of Ute Valley Park. I don't want to disturb them on their breakfast outing. After two hill repeats, I see our neighbor, Steve, in the dark, walking his dog. Then I glimpse the awakening dawn. I am out of breath at the top of the hill. David from the Sunrise

Striders running group is coming down the hill and giving me a thumbs up.

Countdown: 54 Days
Tuesday, September 10, 2019
Colorado Springs, CO

    I feel the cool air on my legs, hands, and entire body. I am out in the pre-dawn light for my 8-mile run. It has been a couple of weeks now of continuous decline in my running speed. I don't seem able to shake off this slowdown in performance. I'm not sure why I've been running slower. Perhaps I need to intensify my speed workouts? Perhaps my legs need a rest with more focus on strength training? I put in nearly 40 miles of running last week. Perhaps I need to focus on short fast runs?

Countdown: 53 Days
Wednesday, September 11, 2019
Colorado Springs, CO

    Today is filled with meetings and is a total-body rest day. I am so fortunate to have a schedule dedicated to running and racing. But I know for certain, even if I were working full time, I would find time to train and race. I love running and it gives back to me more than I ever dreamed possible. I love that running is an individual sport. I don't have to rely on anyone but myself. There are no restrictions on running any time of the day or year. All I need are my running shoes.

Countdown: 52 Days

Thursday, September 12, 2019

Colorado Springs, CO

The weather is beginning to get a bit chilly in the mornings with the temperature in the 50s. As I start on my 12-mile run I am a little cool, but after running for five or 10 minutes I warm up enough to forget about the chill and get into the rhythm of running. I run up the long hill along Flying W Ranch Road and down the other side to N 30th Street, Garden of the Gods Road, and Sinton Trail. I see two other runners on this beautiful crisp morning. Even though it's still dark, I run without my headlamp and become aware of the dawning light on the horizon after a couple of miles. A good training day.

Countdown: 51 Days

Friday, September 13, 2019

Colorado Springs, CO

Today is gym and strength training day. I have been more serious about strength training and yoga than ever before. Craig is running/hiking up to Barr Camp, so he gives me a ride to Accolades Gym at 6:00 on his way to Manitou Springs.

The gym is busy as usual. I meet an older woman, perhaps in her 80s, who tells me she saw me running yesterday on Sinton Trail. I introduce myself to her. Her name is Ellen and she tells me that she has two artificial hips and is not able to run anymore. Hmmm... I see more and more people with replacement parts in their bodies. I find it curious that our bodies can accept foreign materials, such as plastic, titanium, or gold, and be able to function. When I look at nature, everything is perfect, as is. We humans tend to be smart enough to harm our natural environment and ourselves. We hate to endure pain and suffering and yet tend to follow paths that cause more pain and suffering, like lifelong poor diet and exercise habits.

Countdown: 50 Days

Saturday, September 14, 2019

Manitou Springs High School Track, CO

    I do a warmup jog for one mile before getting into my workout, running intervals at the Manitou Springs High School track. The morning air is cool, and the sky is dark. Sunrise is still 40 minutes away. I run a ladder of 4x400m, 2x800m, 1x1mile, then 2x800m, and 4x400m. It's Saturday, the school is closed, and I'm the only person on the track. I love that feeling of having the track all to myself. I always feel fantastic after a hard workout and today is no exception.

Countdown: 49 Days

Sunday, September 15, 2019

Colorado Springs, CO

    I run a 7-mile "joy run" this morning. My Airbnb guest is a yoga instructor, and when I return home, she is ready to practice. I'm a willing Guinea pig, so I pull out two yoga mats and she leads me through a Hatha yoga practice. She is an excellent instructor and corrects my forms. The yoga is very calming, and the stretching feels good after my 7-mile run.

Countdown: 48 Days

Monday, September 16, 2019

Colorado Springs, CO

This morning at 6:00 I run over to Steep Mother and do 10x hill repeats. It is pre-dawn and 40 minutes before sunrise. In the dark, I can make out several deer blocking the entrance to the Ute Valley Park entrance. I make noise—not to scare them, but to alert them to my presence. Fortunately, they move out of the way and head toward the woods, allowing me to run my hill repeats. I hear my name in the dark. It's Steve walking his dog. I complete my workout and cool down with a 3.5-mile run. My hill speed is improved from last week and all repeats are consistent in time.

Countdown: 47 Days

Tuesday, September 17, 2019

Colorado Springs, CO

Tomorrow I have a series of meetings, making it difficult to run early in the morning. Instead, I run eight miles today, in lieu of my gym day. I want to run fast, but somehow I can't find a fast flat 8-mile course around here. Before I went to bed last night, I mapped out in my mind an 8-mile route, not flat, however.

Today I run one warmup mile slightly downhill to the post office. Then I run 1.5 miles uphill along Flying W Ranch Road; it's a grind. I continue one mile down the backside of Flying W Ranch Road, followed by a 1-mile downhill run to Rockrimmon Boulevard and an uphill return. I run one mile past our home to Piñon Valley Park and back home, then back down to Piñon Valley Park, and back home again.

It's not an ideal route for a fast run with the downhills at a faster pace and the uphills at a slower pace, but I work with what I have.

Countdown: 46 Days
Wednesday, September 18, 2019
Colorado Springs, CO

    This morning, at the Pikes Peak Toastmasters club meeting, I give a speech about my Boston Marathon blog. The speech and blog are about the parallels between life and a marathon, and how we face unknowns from the starting line to the finish line. And about the magic of both life and a marathon. I competed against two other speakers and won the best speaker blue ribbon award.

    I am always surprised by how I am becoming a better speaker, and also how much better and more fun my life journey has become. I try to portray kindness and generosity to my running friends by giving them time, two listening ears for their stories of failing to set personal records (PRs), and by making pancakes when they are hungry after a long run. I try to be there for my running friends during their successes and failures. It costs me nothing, and it's been proven that giving returns many benefits to the giver.

Countdown: 45 Days
Thursday, September 19, 2019
Colorado Springs, CO

    My training schedule shows a long, slow 20-mile run today. I am up early and pack my CamelBak with 32 ounces of water and three Spring Energy gels which I discovered recently through my friend, Michelle. Spring Energy gels contain the cleanest ingredients and no animal products. I ate two on my last 18-mile long run and my stomach handled them without any trouble. Today, I'll eat one each at mile 7, mile 12, and mile 17. I start with a slow first mile going easy down Sinton Trail, then connect with the Green Belt Trail which turns into the Santa Fe Trail. I return home via the same route. I complete 20.4 miles at a 10:16 minute/mile pace.

Countdown: 44 Days

Friday, September 20, 2019

Colorado Springs, CO

    I feel a bit tired from yesterday's 20-mile run but do my stretching, upper body, and core workout training as scheduled. I feel perfect after the workout and ready for my tempo run tomorrow before we head to the airport to catch a flight to Billings, MT. Craig's dad has been in an assisted living facility for over two years. The facility is now saying that they are having difficulty moving him around. We are planning to visit alternative facilities in Billings that would be better suited to take care of him. Our body is a vehicle and I plan to take care of mine with exercise and nutritious whole plant food. I don't want to outlive my running days, so I must keep this healthy body moving and running.

Countdown: 43 Days

Saturday, September 21, 2019

Colorado Springs, CO

    I run an early 5-mile run before our drive to the airport.

Craig was born and raised in Billings. Rex, his 94-year-old father, and some other family members still live there. His father is very weak physically, his short-term memory is gone, and he is living completely in the moment. He seems content spending most of his time napping. He never complains about his mobility challenges or anything else for that matter. We will be looking at two facilities with mechanical lifts, which caregivers use to move immobile people around. Our human body is an incredible machine that we must take care of our entire life, not just during any one given period when we are young or old. I plan to take care of my body and treat it like a sacred temple, and it will return good favor, which is health. I want to run, walk, and travel until the end.

Countdown: 42 Days

Sunday, September 22, 2019

Billings, MT

The weather is cooperating while we are in town. Craig booked an Airbnb near asphalt running trails. He is great with the logistics and arrangements of travel. Two blocks from our Airbnb, we run on a beautiful trail that drops down to and follows the Yellowstone River. I find the water very calming. We don't have rivers (just creeks) near our home in Colorado Springs, so whenever I can run along the water, it's a great pleasure and a treat. Not only that, but the altitude in Billings is only 3,123 feet, compared to our home at 6,500 feet. We run with 10% more oxygen in Billings, and I run faster at a sub-9-minute/mile pace. It's fun to run when you don't struggle and have to expend so much effort.

Countdown: 41 Days

Monday, September 23, 2019

<u>Billings, MT</u>

Craig and I run on the same trail we discovered yesterday. I decide to run with more intensity today, and still, I feel much lighter than running in Colorado Spring. We have morning appointments, so we run early in the dark with our headlamps. I see a herd of whitetail deer running and jumping fences. They are spooked by the sound of our footsteps and the light from our headlamps. I try not to startle animals when I'm out running. Luckily, the deer are harmless, and we separate on good terms; no one gets hurt. All living creatures have a right to coexist in harmony with nature.

Countdown: 40 Days

Tuesday, September 24, 2019

<u>Billings, MT</u>

This morning Craig and I explore a different trail in Billings. It's dark and we both wear headlamps again. We see the bright reflecting eyes of three animals in the distance. Craig says he hopes they aren't coyotes. Then I hear a woman's voice, "We're not a pack of coyotes." She is walking three dogs, none of which barked.

Farther on, we discover Chief Black Otter Trail in Swords Park on the Billings Rims overlooking the city. Billings from this view is a beautiful sight in the pre-dawn light.

Countdown: 39 Days

Wednesday, September 25, 2019

<u>Colorado Springs, CO</u>

No running and no workouts today—just a lazy rest day as we travel home.

Countdown: 38 Days

Thursday, September 26, 2019

<u>Colorado Springs, CO</u>

The trail is wet from last night's rain. When I wake up at 5:00 it is still misting with a light wind blowing. I look at my phone for the current local weather, but there is no rain in the forecast. Craig likes to remind me that the most accurate amateur weather forecast can be determined by just looking out the window and checking the temperature of the outside thermometer. As a techie, I blame my phone app for not being accurate. I get up and put on my running clothes, trusting that the mist will soon stop. It's a bit dark out but I'll be running along Centennial Drive, lit by streetlights, for a couple of miles before I reach the unlit Sinton Trail.

The dawn light appears on the horizon when I cross North Chestnut Street on Sinton Trail. I feel light and free this morning without a water bottle or a headlamp. I decide to go out without any great effort for my 12-mile run. When I turn around at the halfway point, I hear my name. I turn and see Sarah from Toastmasters riding a bike with her friend. She zips by me, stops at North Chestnut Street, and we exchange greetings. Running into familiar faces on the trail helps me forget about the exertion of running. It is a strong 12-mile training run for me today.

Countdown: 37 Days

Friday, September 27, 2019

<u>Colorado Springs, CO</u>

I don't feel so great today; my energy level and appetite are low. Perhaps residual fatigue from the Billings trip?

Countdown: 36 Days

Saturday, September 28, 2019

<u>Downtown Colorado Springs, CO</u>

Today is my 64th birthday. My coach asked me to sign up for a long tempo run happening today, a half-marathon race. So here I am downtown, ready to start the Colorado Springs Half Marathon. Colder weather moved in this morning with wind and temperatures in the 50s. With the wind chill, it feels much colder than 50°F. To be honest, I didn't think I would run this morning. Yesterday evening I felt like my head was spinning, an experience that happened to me on one other occasion during a trip to San Diego about 15 years ago. It was scary to have my head spinning and feeling heavy. It didn't matter what position I was in, lying down, standing up, or sitting, I couldn't lift my head. Last night's episode wasn't as severe as the one 15 years ago, but still scary. All I could do was lie down, try to forget about my dizziness, and attempt to sleep.

When I woke up this morning, I felt 100%, so I decided it would be a good day to run the half marathon. Craig takes care of driving and parking. He tells me, "This is your training run. Go out so slow for the first half of the race that you are bored, and then run as fast as you want for the second half. If you run a negative split, you'll feel fast passing other runners during the second half." It's easier said than done since I tend to deplete my energy early by going out hard in a race and then run on fumes in the second half. So, today I am consciously going out slow, chatting with other runners during the early part of the race, and trying to conserve my energy for the latter half. The strategy works out well with a 9:08 minute/mile pace for 13.1 miles. I have the energy to pass other runners in the second half of the race which boosts my confidence. This has never happened in previous races. I run a negative split with a 1:01:03 time at 6.5 miles. Finishing at 1:59:35, I place first out of nine in my age group. At the finish line, I see a familiar face, Richard, who also ran the half marathon. He was also first in his age group and we chatted about our upcoming races.

Countdown: 35 Days
Sunday, September 29, 2019
Colorado Springs, CO

It's a beautiful fall day with sun and a cool wind. I do a cross-training workout at the gym. My body already feels recovered from yesterday's race. I am happy with my good core strength and upper body training today.

Countdown: 34 Days
Monday, September 30, 2019
Colorado Springs, CO

Today is the last day of September and it feels like fall. I run 10x hill repeats in the dark this morning. I have my headlamp on and Steep Mother is familiar to me. I see a couple of people walking their dogs in the dim light. My hill repeats are adequate. I don't set any new uphill records, but I'm consistent, which is okay. My body has been super healthy throughout my New York City Marathon training, and I am so grateful for that.

Countdown: 33 Days

Tuesday, October 1, 2019

<u>Colorado Springs, CO</u>

It is difficult for me to believe that I only have one month of training left before the New York City Marathon. Coach asks me what I'm planning today, and I tell him I'm doing a tempo run. He scolds me by reminding me that I only get three hard workouts per week. I decide to back off and run 6.4 miles in the dark with my headlamp.

I try out my new lightweight marathon shoes that arrived by mail a couple of days earlier. It's a good idea to try them before my 20-mile run on Thursday and a good idea to run 20 miles in them before I run 26.2 miles in them during the marathon. Sure enough, my heel is tight up against my socks and I stop after three miles to re-tie my shoelaces. I avoid getting a blister and my training run is only okay. I have to accept the fact that not every day will be a perfect training day. There will be some good ones, some not-so-good ones, and some surprisingly great training runs. That's the nature of any training cycle.

I carry my phone and listen to the ChiRunning app to help me work on my running form. While listening to the app, a coach constantly describes how to align my posture, my arm swings, my pelvic rotation, and my head position, all with a metronome to keep my cadence at 180 steps per minute. My mind wanders during my run, and soon I hear the coach repeating the same instructions, bringing me back into focus on my form. I enjoy using the app and wish that I had learned about it sooner.

Countdown: 32 Days
Wednesday, October 2, 2019
Colorado Springs, CO

After my workout at the gym, I soak in the hot sauna. Sometimes it feels so good just to sit in the sauna and breathe deeply.

Countdown: 31 Days
Thursday, October 3, 2019
Colorado Springs, CO

I run 20 miles. It is dark and foggy and feels cold. I start at 5:30 with a headlamp, one energy gel, one electrolyte gel, and 18 ounces of water. I begin running slowly to conserve my energy for the later miles. I pass a few more runners than usual as I head down Sinton Trail and up the Greenbelt Trail connecting to the Santa Fe Trail. I turn around at ten miles. Eating the electrolyte gel with water is good, giving me hydration and energy, but when I take the energy gel at mile 13 my side starts to cramp. I hang on to my side with one hand and slow my pace. After a few minutes, the cramp disappears. Thank goodness. I have a decent long-distance training run. I notice my pace is 16 seconds/mile slower on the same route as compared to my March 19th, 20-mile Boston Marathon training run.

Countdown: 30 Days
Friday, October 4, 2019
<u>Colorado Springs, CO</u>

    I rest today.

Countdown: 29 Days
Saturday, October 5, 2019
<u>Glenwood Springs, CO</u>

    We plan to drive to Aspen, Colorado for a colorful fall-foliage weekend getaway. Of course, the fall colors in Colorado are no comparison to fall colors in New England. The New England colors are so vibrant and amazing, it feels like heaven on earth when you drive down the road. The New England roads are gradually covered with freshly dropped leaves, and when you walk over them, you can hear them quietly speaking to you. These thoughts bring back many fall memories of New England and Maine where I lived for many years and of New England roads nearly completely shaded by large deciduous trees. You can hardly see the sky through the colorful fall leaves. After my eight half-mile intervals, we pack our lunch and head out for our short getaway, enjoying the freedom and the fall. We stay in an Airbnb in Dillon for the night.

Countdown: 28 Days
Sunday, October 6, 2019
<u>Glenwood Springs, CO</u>

    Craig and I run from the Two Rivers Park in Glenwood Springs on a trail toward Aspen along the Roaring Fork

River. It feels like ChiRunning with the calming energy of the river, the trees, and the sun all in sync moving my feet forward. It's an exploratory run, which is fun. Somehow Craig is passing me at mile five, flying down the trail. I finish mile six right behind him.

After the run, we soak in Glenwood Hot Springs. Neither Craig nor I are people who can soak in hot water for a long time and after 40 minutes we're done. After the hot springs, we drive from Glenwood Springs to Aspen and see the most animated orange, yellow, and red fall colors surrounded by deep, dark greens. There isn't enough time to drive to Maroon Bells, but we eat an organic, plant-based lunch at the Spring Cafe in Aspen. We are really happy to find the Spring Cafe since our favorite Pyramid Bistro restaurant is closed for the season. Surprisingly, we find even better meal choices for us at the Spring Cafe.

Countdown: 27 Days

Monday, October 7, 2019

Colorado Springs, CO

Today I run 10x hill repeats up Steep Mother. It's still dark at 6:20 but light enough to run uphill on this familiar terrain, knowing that soon the sun will rise. I can always count on the sun rising, no matter what. Is there anything else in life that is so predictable and consistent? I run into Lu and Steve with their dog. There are many deer on the trail who look at me as if asking, "What are you doing?" or "Why are you breathing so hard?" as they jump to the side. I respond, "Hi guys, how are you doing today?"

After I finish my hill repeats, I do a cooldown run on Seven Oaks Drive. I hear someone yelling my name and saying hello. It's Julie from Toastmasters, walking. It is a very pleasant surprise to see her this morning.

Countdown: 26 Days

Tuesday, October 8, 2019

Colorado Springs, CO

My training schedule calls for an 8-mile run tomorrow, but since I have a 6:44 meeting, I decide to run the eight miles today. I love to run first thing in the morning. Running later in the day often means time constraints due to other commitments.

I seemed to have plateaued in my running speed. My legs feel tired but, with my new Altra Escalante shoes laced up properly today, they fit much better and my feet feel good. When I start my run, the weather is perfect and at mile five the wind starts to pick up. I think this is exactly like running in New York City—cold and always into the wind! Nature is trying to teach me that weather is one element I don't have control over and that I just need to deal with it. What other choice is there than going with the flow of nature?

Countdown: 25 Days

Wednesday, October 9, 2019

Colorado Springs, CO

I attend my 6:44 Toastmasters meetings. I am passionate about improving my public speaking and growing my leadership skills. After the club meeting today, we have an officers' meeting. I don't pay much attention to the meeting and feel like time is being wasted when some officers keep chatting about nothing important, not making any points, and not adding value to the meeting. After the meeting, I go to the gym and work out.

Countdown: 24 Days
Thursday, October 10, 2019
<u>Colorado Springs, CO</u>

It is windy and snowy. The first storm of the season has arrived and gives me a glimpse of what's to come. I start running at 6:40, heading north, with the wind hammering my face and body. The wind is so strong that I feel like it's pushing me backward. I hunker my face down and keep going but I'm losing the battle with nature this morning. I decide to turn around at one mile and go south with the wind. Guess what, it's a lot easier to run with the wind pushing at my back. This feels like ChiRunning, going with nature's energy and power. This is the first time this fall that I run with my winter face mask, winter hat, and warm gloves, the perfect choice for today's weather. I tough it out and complete 12 miles of running in the wind and snow.

Countdown: 23 Days
Friday, October 11, 2019
<u>Colorado Springs, CO</u>

With less than a month to go before I position myself behind the starting line of the New York Marathon, I download my marathon confirmation form containing my bib number: 46101, Orange Wave 3, and Corral D. I just read a blog on the marathon website providing information on the pre-start wait on Staten Island. The blog suggests making friends, bringing warm clothes for the three-plus-hour wait, and taking it easy on the free bagels and coffee.

I look at the course elevation profile map for the first time and discover that the course is not entirely flat. The first mile has a 160-foot climb up one side of the Verrazano-Narrows Bridge connecting Staten Island to Brooklyn with the second mile down the other side of the bridge. Then the course has small ups and downs. From mile 14.5 to mile 15.5, we will climb 100 feet up to the top of the Queensboro Bridge. A 65-foot elevation gain awaits us at mile 23 (yikes) at Fifth Avenue. Although a 65-foot elevation gain doesn't sound like a lot, it comes late in the race and I know I'll feel it. It looks like a tough enough course to me, which means it will require plenty of patience and preparation.

Countdown: 22 Days

Saturday, October 12, 2019

<u>Manitou Springs High School Track, CO</u>

Today is my last track workout before the New York City Marathon. I wake up and look at the results of Eliud Kipchoge's 26.2-mile run in Vienna, Austria with a challenge to beat two hours. The event took place eight hours ago while I was peacefully sleeping. I predicted his time at 1:59:42, and I see he finished at 1:59:40. What an amazing person, not only as a runner but for who he is. He has amazing mental discipline. He once stated, "Discipline is doing what's right, not doing what you feel like." And one of his famous quotes I live by is "No human is limited."

I'm a good example of this credo. I never ran my entire life until 2011 and just look how far I've come. The human body and mind are incredible when both are working together. Eliud Kipchoge is my hero and inspiration. Motivated, I give it my all during my track workout this morning. It is an outstanding workout.

Countdown: 21 Days

Sunday, October 13, 2019

Colorado Springs, CO

It is a beautiful, cool morning to run a few miles. I run up Flying W Ranch Road with 350 feet of elevation gain and a drop of 300 feet to 30th Street on the other side of Mountain Shadows Pass. I return the way I came, climbing up 300 feet, then running down 350 feet. I start running in the dark and after one mile I see day breaking on the horizon. Deer are looking at me with curiosity as if wondering why I'm up and running so early. Magpies are always up yakking amongst themselves. I hear the owls hooting. I usually spot owls by their glowing eyes but am unable to locate their eyes in the dark this morning. A skunk is on the trail too, and I do not want to get tangled up with that. I know the scent from skunks is used to make the most expensive perfumes, but the unaltered odor is a different matter. I'm not into processed scents. The scent of my sweat is enough to get me into the shower after my runs.

Countdown: 20 Days

Monday, October 14, 2019

Colorado Springs, CO

It has been quite a weekend of accomplishments from Kipchoge's 1:59:40 26.2 mile run to the marathon times of familiar runners in the 2019 Chicago Marathon. I am so pumped up for my New York City Marathon run. The air temperature this morning is warmer than it has been in the last couple of weeks. I run my last 10x hill repeats. I feel strong and consistent with each of the uphill runs under 1:40. This week I will run my last long, 20-mile training run before I taper for the marathon.

Countdown: 19 Days

Tuesday, October 15, 2019

<u>Colorado Springs, CO</u>

When I wake up and look at the clock, it's 6:20. How did this happen? I can't believe I slept in. I always wake up at 5:00. The only activity I did yesterday that could have tired me out was hill repeats. I leave the house at 7:20 after eating a piece of toast and drinking a cup of coffee. I run my usual route backward today, down Bourke Drive to Mule Deer, and 30th Street to Flying W Ranch Road to climb up the hill. I feel really good today. After my 7-mile run, I work in the garden and dig up some overgrown Russian sage plants. The Russian sages are very hardy in this harsh Colorado environment. They grow without much water and, since deer won't eat them, they thrive. After a couple of hours of work I have the front flower garden cleaned up. I will clean up the gardens in the backyard when I return from the marathon. With my taper, I don't want to use too much of my energy on the gardens.

Countdown: 18 Days

Wednesday, October 16, 2019

Colorado Springs, CO

    I spend the morning at the gym doing some light strength training and stretching.

Countdown: 17 Days

Thursday, October 17, 2019

Colorado Springs, CO

    Today is my last 20-mile run before the New York City Marathon. I'm up early but don't feel quite 100%. I set my mind to the task and start running anyway, with my fuel gels and 32 ounces of water in my CamelBak. I finish my 20-miles but don't feel like I would have been able to push on to 26.2 miles.

Countdown: 16 Days

Friday, October 18, 2019

Colorado Springs, CO

    I am down with a cough and runny nose. My body is telling me that I need to stay in bed. I rest and do strength training at home.

Countdown: 15 Days

Saturday, October 19, 2019

Colorado Springs, CO

    I run a personal-best half-mile during my interval training today. Even though my body is under attack, I gave it my best for my training run. I don't have much time left before the marathon.

Countdown: 14 Days

Sunday, October 20, 2019

<u>Colorado Springs, CO</u>

    I work out at the gym but am still under the weather. My body needs more rest. I stay in bed after my workout and get up every two hours for something to drink and eat. I drink my cold-fighting tea of hot water, sage, lemon, and honey.

Countdown: 13 Days

Monday, October 21, 2019

<u>Colorado Springs, CO</u>

    I have been down for the past 72 hours following my 20-mile run on Thursday. Perhaps it was the cold air I was breathing as I ran. It's only 12 days until the marathon. I run 6x hill repeats with my worst times. I've trained all year for this marathon. These hill-repeat times should have been my best.

    I finish my training, eat some warm oatmeal, and go back to bed for another four hours of rest. During the day, I use up an entire box of Kleenex for my runny nose. I don't want hugs or handshakes from anyone right now. I know my immune system is strong, but my body has been working hard during my training and is perhaps a bit run down. I need to get to the starting line in my healthiest state, both mentally and physically.

Countdown: 12 Days
Tuesday, October 22, 2019

Colorado Springs, CO

I can hardly breathe after sitting in the sauna at the gym for 30 minutes. The sweat is pouring out of me. I'm hopeful that the sauna will cleanse the bugs from my body. I look at my training schedule. Even though I'm feeling physically down, I haven't missed any training runs since last Friday. I expect to be 100% tomorrow and go for a run and will hope the mental calm from running provides relief from my physical illness.

Countdown: 11 Days
Wednesday, October 23, 2019

Colorado Springs, CO

Okay, it is only eleven days until the marathon and I am still not feeling 100%. I wasn't being honest with myself when I got up this morning, told myself I was better, and ran five miles. Yikes. Not the best plan. Okay body, you are telling me you are not 100%. This would have been the time to listen to my coach when he gently told me to give myself one more day of rest. But do I ever listen to anyone, coach included? I ran anyway and now I'm discouraged and disappointed. I should be in peak shape this week. You should rest when you're not feeling well. I can easily say those words to my running friends, but when it comes to me, it's dang hard to do it. I feel like a moron. After my disappointing run, I go to the gym and soak in the sauna. Honestly, though, I think I'm beginning to feel better.

Countdown: 10 Days

Thursday, October 24, 2019

<u>Colorado Springs, CO</u>

I'm still down for another day from my cold. Last night I worked at setting an intention for my cold to depart 100%. My coughing is subdued and my runny nose is almost dry, two really good signs of recovery. I want to fully rest today instead of following my running taper schedule. Yes, I have finally realized that it would be in my best interest to stay in, instead of doing my scheduled 10-mile run. I still have tomorrow, Saturday, and Sunday to make up the training runs, so I think I'll be okay. Life is all about how to handle unexpected challenges, curveballs, and adjusting when necessary.

Countdown: 9 Days

Friday, October 25, 2019

<u>Colorado Springs, CO</u>

The countdown to the marathon is now in the single digits. I am still down. I sit in the sauna at the gym, but perhaps even that's not a good idea since it's sucking up all my energy. I come home and research the effects of hot saunas on a cold. It seems to help, according to the research so maybe it was not a bad plan, but I don't know how it will help me recover any quicker.

Countdown: 8 Days

Saturday, October 26, 2019

Colorado Springs, CO

I sauna at the gym, walk two miles and feel good. I come home and go to bed. No long run today and perhaps no more running days before the marathon.

Countdown: 7 Days

Sunday, October 27, 2019

Colorado Springs, CO

Today is the day. I must feel 100% by the end of the day or I might have to consider not running the New York City Marathon. If I choose not to run this year, I'll have other opportunities. It's not like missing out on the Olympic Trials, which only come once every four years. It would be difficult to stomach the idea of not running after all these days and months of training, but I know my body will tell me what to do when the time comes.

Countdown: 6 Days

Monday, October 28, 2019

Colorado Springs, CO

My body is still telling me to do nothing except rest, rest, and REST even more.

Countdown: 5 Days

Tuesday, October 29, 2019

<u>Colorado Springs, CO</u>

Today I feel a lot better. Thank you, universe.

It has been snowing all day. It's like the snows I remember in Maine, coming steadily down, hour after hour, under dark clouds. The accumulation will make workers' commutes challenging and cause many cancellations. I feel like my body has been through a similar storm. I have not run one inch since last Wednesday and I have been down for 12 days. Now I have to decide if I give up on the New York City marathon or not. Perhaps I should just visit family instead. My sisters in South Korea, who don't know anything about running or marathons, ask me why I run and what the medals mean to me at this stage of my life. I don't have clear answers to those questions.

Countdown: 4 Days

Wednesday, October 30, 2019

<u>Colorado Springs, CO</u>

My body is not healing. As I continue to worry about my slow recovery and not being able to taper my running properly, I put myself under more stress. This is the first time that I am fighting against the clock. I know I can't win against time, but I keep trying anyway.

Countdown: 3 Days

Thursday, October 31, 2019

Colorado Springs, CO

I continue to rest, rest, and rest more, though I don't feel much improvement from yesterday.

Countdown: 2 Days

Friday, November 1, 2019

Colorado Springs, CO

I feel good enough to make the trip to New York City. I hope that with a couple of days left before the marathon, I will completely recover and be able to run. I am no longer coughing, and my runny nose has dried up. I am hopeful.

We leave the house at 8:15 a.m. and drive to the Denver airport for our direct flight to New York's LaGuardia airport. Craig booked us into an Airbnb in Manhattan, close to the marathon bus loading location at Bryant Park. Craig and I arrive in Manhattan around 6:00 p.m. Craig is hungry and finds a Whole Foods Market around the corner from our Airbnb. I don't have an appetite so Craig goes by himself. I rest with my hot water, lemon, and honey.

Countdown: 1 Day

Saturday, November 2, 2019

New York City, NY

I hope for the strength to run a 3-mile shakeout run today. It doesn't happen. Craig runs out to Central Park and comes back with a big smile telling me how much is going on and about seeing all the runners out for a shakeout run. I am in the bed, feeling sorry for myself. My body is not coming around. I was so wrong. I had thought by now that I would be feeling like a runner again and ready for the marathon, but my body is still giving the idea a big thumbs down.

We plan to spend time with our two-year-old granddaughter, Aria, after the marathon. If I run, I could further stress my body, have a cold relapse, and risk being quarantined from Aria. I don't want my young granddaughter to get what I have been carrying for the last two weeks. I wouldn't wish this cold on anyone.

Around 7:00 p.m., Craig shows me the marathon cancellation policy. I have until midnight to cancel my entry and have a guaranteed entry for next year. With much apprehension, I log into my marathon account and click the cancellation button. I feel a sense of loss and at the same time, relief. All the worry about not being healthy enough to run and then not being able to spend time with my granddaughter has suddenly disappeared. I text my children with my decision not to run. They all support my decision, although my coach is disappointed. This is the first time all year that I haven't been able to stand at the starting line for a race. Now I understand how others feel who don't get to start a race for whatever reasons or those who start a race and are unable to finish.

Even though I worship my body as a sacred temple, sometimes it sends me a signal to alter my plans. The lesson I've learned is that I can never be careful enough when it comes to taking care of myself. What a disappointment. Right now, I think I may never run again. I've been through this before, though, a few years ago when I got injured during a run and swore off running. The wound healed quickly into a gravity tattoo and I have hardly missed a beat or a run since then.

Countdown: 0 Day
Sunday, November 3, 2019
<u>New York City, NY</u>

Do I need to get up this morning?

My wonderful husband and coach makes me oatmeal for breakfast and suggests we go out and watch the marathon. We are staying about two blocks from mile 16, and Craig calculates the elite runners will begin coming by at 10:30, so we have time to visit St. Patrick's Cathedral before hand. It seems appropriate to go to the Cathedral for my sanity and a bit of peace. It's only a few blocks from where we are staying, and I need to move. I have never taken so many days off from either walking or running. It is a perfect opportunity to take my mind off the disappointment of not running the marathon.

St. Patrick's Cathedral is considered a symbol of Roman Catholicism in New York. The place is filled with visitors and congregation members who are there for the Sunday Service. Afterward, on our walk to mile 16, I decided to stop in a coffee shop. I have been avoiding caffeine for two weeks preparing for my coffee/caffeine performance boost on race day. Well, now I can have a coffee guilt-free since I'm not running today.

I enjoy my coffee while waiting for the first runners to come by. There are so many people out cheering. A band is playing continuously. I feel the race energy and when I see the first group of elite runners, I scream like a crazy woman. There are a lot of wheelchair participants coming by. They are amazingly fast. Now we see a few elite women along with fast men. We watch runners until we go back to our Airbnb for lunch.

Making the best out of the day under the circumstances, after lunch, Craig and I decide to visit the 9/11 memorial. On our way to the memorial, we walk through Korea Town, a first for Craig. Oh, how I miss Korean food. I eat the hot kimchi stew knowing that it will knock the final socks off my cold. Craig is laying on his Korean language skills to the Korean servers. Every time Craig says, "It's delicious," and "Thank you" in Korean, the servers smile. We both fill our stomachs with hot stew and continue our walk to the 9/11 memorial. I visited the site when the building construction started but have not been there since. The site evokes so much emotion. Seeing the monument with the names of those who fell on that fateful day is powerful and inspires much introspection. The memorial building has integrated some portions of the original twin tower foundation pieces into it. It has a surreal effect and echoes my emotions today.

2020

New Attempt

January 2020

Colorado Springs

I have visited the New York City Marathon website (https://www.nyrr.org/tcsnycmarathon) many times. Today when I click it open to apply for the 2020 New York City Marathon, I feel calm, like an experienced runner who's done this before, and yet excited to be applying for this prestigious race again. Because I canceled my entry the night before the 2019 New York City Marathon, when I input my information today, I get an immediate notification that I am accepted! How many people get a second chance at the Big One? Plus, now I have another year to train. I feel a sense of gratitude and privilege to get another chance at this marathon. Life is nothing but new attempts. With every new breath I am born again, and with each new day, my journey begins anew. The variables—weather, logistics, runners, physical shape, mindset—continually flow and change. All I can hope for is to progress and learn from previous experiences. "Progress equals happiness" according to Tony Robbins.

Hopeful*
February 2020
<u>*Colorado Springs*</u>

Although the New York City Marathon is ten months away, I have been training and participating in local races since the beginning of the year—Rescue Run 10k, Winter Series (four races, each two weeks apart, progressively longer in distance), and the Super Half Marathon. I also ran the McAllen, Texas marathon between two Winter Series races. The Winter Series races are put on by the Pikes Peak Road Runners (PPRR)—a local, 46-year-old, 1500-member running club. The mission of the PPRR is to promote running and personal fitness, and I feel honored to be a member. The club is inclusive of anyone willing to join, and it is fun and relaxing to run with others also training for the upcoming race season. I have been a member since

2012 and love seeing all the runners and familiar faces that show up for the races and training events. This year I decided to run the short Winter Series races (3-mile, 4-mile, 5-mile, and 10-km) to supplement my speed workouts in preparation for the Seoul International Marathon in March. My training goal is to stay upright on the sometimes icy, muddy racecourses and finish strong and healthy. And I did. I placed first in the Rescue Run, Super Half, and McAllen Marathon. I finished second in the Winter Series.

Detour!

March 2020

Little Rock, Arkansas

Spoiler alert! Last year my coach, Craig, won the lottery drawing into the March 1st, 2020 Tokyo Marathon. Then comes reality. Rumors were beginning in January through February of concerns about a new virus in China, but no one could imagine the impact on our so-called normal lives.

This month, the World Health Organization (WHO) declared the novel coronavirus (COVID-19) outbreak a global pandemic. The pandemic spread worldwide like wildfire and changed our plans and lives forever. Due to this virus, travel restrictions and lockdowns, the official Tokyo Marathon cancellation came via email in the middle of February. We scrambled to cancel our Asia trip plans including my Seoul International Marathon scheduled for March 22nd and a visit with my family in South Korea. Before that, Craig and I had been debating overseas travel. Craig was willing to travel, but I was hesitant to talk to him about my concerns. Thankfully, I didn't have to voice my worries since the decision was made by the

Tokyo Marathon officials. With Craig in peak condition for a March 1st marathon, he quickly looked for a domestic race and found the Little Rock Marathon in Arkansas. I understand him wanting to take advantage of his hard training. We both end up in Little Rock on March 1st. Since I am three weeks behind Craig in training, I sign up for the half marathon.

The weather is perfect with the temperature in the 50s and overcast skies. The start time of 8:00 and the start line location are the same for both races, perfect for us. I run with Craig for a mile before Craig says, "This is your half, tear it up." I took off. I was already at the 7-mile turnaround point when I saw Craig at about 6.5-miles. I came in 1st out of 82 in my age group with a time of 1:55:11, and a pace of 8:47 minutes/mile (when Mira, my daughter, received the results by text, she replied, "Holy shit ma"). I went to the massage tent. The line was long, but I knew I had plenty of time before Craig would finish the marathon.

Starting at 3 hours and 30 minutes, my eyes are glued to the big screen in the convention center showing a live stream of the runners crossing the finish line. As each minute goes by, I wonder if I missed him. At noon, it has been four hours since the start, and he should be here by now. I don't take my eyes off the monitor. Finally, he crosses the line with a time of 4:30:38. He looks good and walks slowly toward me. He took his sweet time to finish this one. He seems happy with his finish although he was in top shape and his training runs may have suggested a faster time. The weather was ideal, and I anticipated him finishing earlier. Then again, sometimes that's just how it unfolds.

They have a wonderful indoor finisher's venue with tables and chairs and indoor bathrooms. The finisher's medal must weigh ten pounds (only a slight exaggeration). We left our medals at our Airbnb since we didn't want to carry around the extra weight in our continuing travels. The Airbnb host's child enjoyed playing with the medals.

Craig and I had never been to Arkansas, Tennessee, or Mississippi, so we decide to visit those states during this trip. Also, I wanted to soak up some warm weather. So after the race and touring those three states, we fly to Florida for some warm weather. We fly home from Miami on March 13th as national COVID-19 concerns become more acute.

Solo

April 2020

<u>Colorado Springs</u>

Looking out our home office window I see six inches of new snow! Our backyard adjoins Ute Valley Park and the 156-foot bluff on the west side of the park. The scenery is serene and peaceful. I did a long run yesterday (a half marathon, 13.1 miles) in anticipation of last night's snowfall. From our front door, I ran a mile north on our neighborhood trail following Vindicator Drive and Rockrimmon Blvd before heading south on the Pikes Peak Greenway Trail. I then ran up Sinton Trail from Monument Creek and back home. For two-thirds of my run, the trails were adjacent to flowing creeks. Listening to and watching the water flow is a life lesson to me about speed and direction—steady, without effort, and always downhill. For a portion of my run along the creek, I am running downhill in the same direction as the flowing water. It feels easy and without effort going with the flow.

I'm surprised when I see John, from the Sunrise Striders running group, at mile 3. Usually, this time of year, I would be running in Garden of the Gods Park with the Sunrise Striders. Due to COVID-19 and social distancing, we are all running solo. I'm fortunate to live close to many trails with plenty of route options and enjoy an easy run without any time pressure. At mile 12, I see Michelle and her running buddy. We are all doing our social distancing duty to minimize virus exposure and transmission.

Although all major races are currently canceled, later in the month, I run a "virtual" (solo) race put on by the Demoor Global Running Group. My wonderful coach drops me off in Monument, Colorado, 13.1 miles uphill from the Woodmen Road Santa Fe trailhead. The sun is rising with a breeze blowing in my face. I start running easily and without stress or competing runners. It is a personal best (and first) virtual run with a finish time of 2:06:42 and a pace of 9:39 minutes/mile. How sweet it is to be greeted with a big smile from my coach, the only person at the finish line.

Course Correction

May 2020

Colorado Springs

Although the infection rate numbers are subsiding following the earlier exponential growth of COVID-19 cases, cancellations keep showing up on race websites. As part of my regular training, I run three half marathon distances in May, logging one of my highest monthly mileage in my Garmin training log—miles: 173.8, time: 35:39:29, calories: 13,286 C. It's funny that Garmin is so stingy about the number of calories I burn per running mile. It gives me 70 calories per mile. I feel like I am burning at least 90 calories per mile, in my humble mind.

May is my favorite time of the year. In May, every corner of the landscape turns lime green, expressing innocence, youth, and freshness with everything coming back to life after winter. Inhaling the sweet smell of Russian Olive trees and the pleasing smells of lilac blooms along the trail puts me in a state of "awe." I am reminded of nature's gift, the new bloom of life that I have ignored for more than half my life. It is an awaking as I now try to take in all that nature has to offer, every time. What is this life about? We are born helpless and require our parents' unconditional love and care. Then we go into the uncertain teenage years, followed by wrestling with our choices of education and intimate relationships. As life progresses, we continue the struggle by raising kids and pursuing a career during the prime of our lives. Then, we might realize that we didn't center our attention on what matters most in life and attempt to correct our course in mid-life. We must, first and foremost, focus on our health. As my mom always said, "Health is wealth." It's why I now center my life on health, spending more time with family, serving others, and enjoying my newfound passion for running. Life is somewhat like running a marathon. As we run each mile, we tune in to see how our body and mind are performing. "Do I need to drink more water, replenish my fuel, or run faster (slower)?" It's smart to make adjustments at each moment and each mile. Crossing a finish line without regrets brings me a feeling of triumph. As I move forward in life, I try to live without any new regrets before crossing that ultimate finish line.

COVID-19

June 2020

<u>Mount Rushmore, South Dakota</u>

I open my email from the New York City Marathon official. They are canceling the 50th New York City Marathon due to COVID-19. I think my heart stops for several seconds. Although I'm not surprised by the announcement, I had a tiny amount of hope that the race would still happen since we were four months away—enough time, I thought, for the COVID-19 situation to improve. And yet, the decision is the responsible one and I accept it. I understand the enormity of the potential consequences of gatherings of more than fifty thousand runners, fifty thousand volunteers, and millions of spectators. Many races are being canceled, and yet I have been faithfully training—doing my interval speed workouts, my hill repeats, and my weekly long runs, running 35 to 40 miles per week, as if the races are still on. I am a disciplined athlete, and therefore know that my efforts aren't wasted. I'm building my running base and endurance, just like my competitors who are also always training.

I realize the training has been fun without the pressure of in-person races. I am improving my form and speed with the freedom of not having to achieve a target time and distance, just confident that when I am on the starting line of a race, I am stronger and faster than in the previous race. My philosophy is all about progress and growing in every single part of my life. I strive to improve my strength, time, distance, and life in general. At the beginning of the month, I participated in a four-person virtual marathon relay race. I was assigned to three team members from all over the world and we finished 2,695th place out of 11,465. Craig and

I were vacationing in Rapid City, South Dakota when I ran this virtual race starting in Founders Park on a trail along Rapid Creek. He encouraged me along my 6.55 miles, and I finished in 58:47 minutes with an 8:58 minute/mile pace. I was so happy to push hard in this race, running only with Craig pulling me along.

I am an opportunist during the lockdown period, using the time to climb some of the spectacular Colorado mountains and do some mountain biking. Colorado is famous for its 53 mountain peaks over fourteen thousand feet above sea level (14ers). Some would say there are 58 14ers, but others make the distinction that to be a fourteen-thousand-foot peak, "a peak must rise at least 300 feet above the saddle that connects it to the nearest 14er (if another exists nearby)." I have climbed and run portions of Pikes Peak several times during training and have run the Pikes Peak Ascent race twice. Craig and I have the 14er bug, and this month we summit Quandary Peak (14,265 ft) with an elevation gain of 3,450 feet and a roundtrip distance of 6.75 miles from the trailhead. The hike up is a grind and most of the trail is not runnable (for me). When I reach the summit, however, it is hard to explain the feeling of beauty, freedom, and accomplishment.

Nature's Way

July 2020

Buena Vista, Colorado

The uncertainty surrounding COVID-19 continues as I look for a message from the Chicago Marathon race officials. The race is scheduled for October 11th and still, no final decision has been made. I know the announcement will come soon.

We plan to summit Mt. Shavano (14,229 ft) the Monday after the 4th of July, cross the saddle (dropping more than 300 feet), and climb up to Tabegauch Peak (14,155 ft). The night before the climb, we stay 45 minutes from the trailhead, in Salida, a town that comes alive in the summer with white water rafting on the Arkansas River. We watch the weather report and get up at 3:45 to allow us to summit and return to the trailhead before noon, ahead of the potential afternoon thunderstorms. After oatmeal and a hot cup of organic coffee, we drive to the trailhead in the dark and begin our hike at 5:15, the crack of dawn, making our headlamps unnecessary. We checked out the trailhead the day before and are familiar with the first mile of the trail. There are cars in the parking lot, indicating there may be a few hikers ahead of us. As usual, Craig starts running up the trail and I try not to lose sight of him. But soon, I am alone in the quiet light of daybreak. I overtake three young hikers after two miles and one says to me, "Your husband said to pick up the pace… just don't shoot the messenger." I said okay and smiled at them, feeling some comfort knowing hikers are behind me and I am setting the pace. The three young men don't catch up with me until I reached the second summit (Tabegauche Peak). I catch up with Craig at the summit of the first peak, Mt. Shavano, scrabbling through giant boulders in the calm breeze. There is a hikers' party at the summit complete with big smiles, delicious snacks, and hikers' stories. After strenuously hiking for several hours, all food tastes wonderful.

I saw a few strong runners, running up to the peak and back down. Very few sections of the trail are runnable for me, but I ran where I could. As you might imagine on a mountain made of stone, there were many beautiful rocks. I kept picking one up only to drop it and exchange it for the next colorful rock. Is that just human nature? Once you find something you love, you should keep it, but we tend to compare and constantly desire something better.

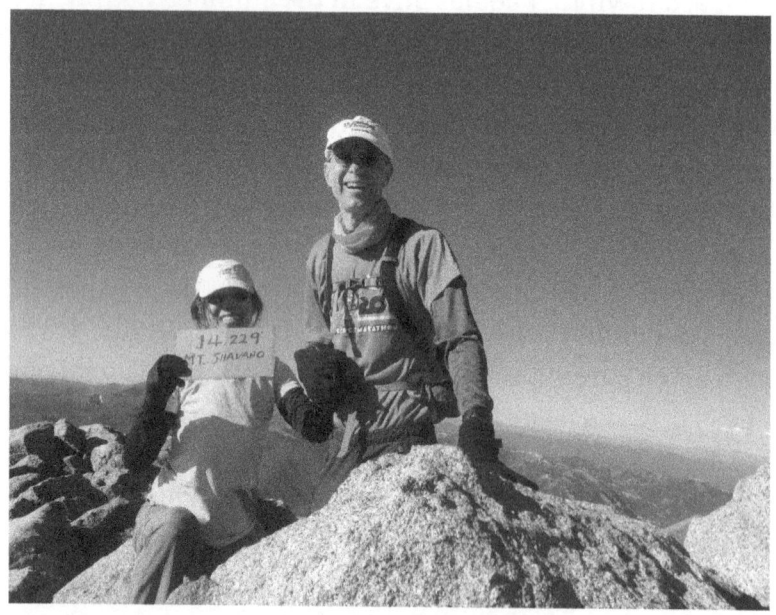

Atop Mount Shavano

The next weekend we drive to Lake City, Colorado, and check into the North Face Lodge for a good night's rest before summiting Redcloud Peak (14,034 ft) and Sunshine Peak (14,001 ft). That night it feels like we are getting ready for a big race as we lay out our shoes, socks, clothes, water bottles, fuel, sunscreen, and headlamp. The drive to the trailhead the next morning is rough with rockslides, potholes, and only one lane in some parts of the road. A single mishap could spell, "Game Over," with a drop off the side of the mountain. Fortunately, Craig is familiar with these driving conditions having grown up driving in the Montana mountains. We arrive at the nearly full trailhead and find some people camped in the parking lot. We see a few lights from hikers' headlamps as we start in the dark at 5:06 with our own headlamps illuminating the trail. Soon we are crossing bubbling creeks as the dawn light turns the skies blue. The wind is calm. The ineffable views from the summits were filled with snowcapped mountains as far as the eye could see. The trail reminds me of hiking from Crested Butte to Aspen with the music of the creek flowing and the colorful wildflowers—Colorado blue columbine, bluebells, and Indian paintbrush.

Our next memorable climb the following week is to the summit of Mount Belford (14,197 ft) and Mount Oxford (14,153 ft) from the Missouri Gulch trailhead 15 miles from our stay in Buena Vista. We get up at 2:00, eat our oatmeal and coffee, leave the motel at 3:00, and arrive at the trailhead at 3:45. Periodically during the beginning of the hike, we turn off our headlamps and gaze at the many stars. Jupiter guides us up the trail. At half a mile, Craig and I pass a young couple who we don't see again until we are on our way down. They are two hours behind us. The backside of Mount Belford on the way to Mount Oxford is brutal with steep, rocky slopes. I am on my hands and knees for a portion of this hike. The summit of Mount Oxford is cool with a gentle breeze. The view of snowcapped Mount Harvard and Mount Missouri is grand. I feel all alone with the soothing sound of the creek and brightly colored flowers. I see fireweeds and many other flowers with names foreign to my vocabulary. They are all unique and beautiful individually, and together they create a dazzling canvas only nature can paint.

Nature offers me peace and a chance to completely forget everything happening back at home. With every footstep, I experience the earth through my body. Nature has so much to offer humans. The birds, rocks, trees, wildflowers, and wild animals are not concerned about COVID-19. Nature is living and thriving as it normally does and welcoming more humans during this unusual time. Nature greets us as if to say, "It's about time you figured this out and enjoyed the perfect earth." It is a reminder that everything is as it should be—it is "nature's way."

Mountains are Calling

August 2020

Winter Park, Colorado

    August arrives with hope and excitement. Winter Park, Colorado is hosting a half marathon and 5 km race. Craig and I sign up right away. It has been a racing drought for us since completing the Little Rock, Arkansas marathon and half marathon in March. This course is mostly on gravel roads and trails with plenty of elevation gain (and loss). We show up at the starting line with our masks on to pick up our race bibs. I am in the first wave of ten runners. We start right at 8:00 and for the first mile we seem to be chasing black Angus cows through a meadow. I try to avoid slippery cow pies on the trail. After the meadow, all ten of us turn onto a road. I hear some runners say, "I think we're going the wrong way." I turn around and run back while others continue in the wrong direction. I finally see where we should have gone straight rather than turning left. Yay, I'm back on course. The route is a grueling uphill climb, especially mile six on a single-track dirt trail with piles of rocks. After mile seven, we make a lollipop circle and head downhill breathing more comfortably. At mile nine I am struggling and need an energy gel, but all I'm carrying is water. My stomach starts aching and I keep telling myself, "You got this. You can run four more miles." I fight off fatigue during the last mile and finally cross the finish line with a time of 2:25:27. Surprisingly, Craig has been at the finish line for a while. He had a good run with a time of 2:01:07. I won my age group and finish 31st out of 44 runners. Three runners DNF'd (did not finish). It was a tough but beautiful course. The race has revitalized my running spirit, if only for a day.

 I start a once-a-month run up Pikes Peak Barr Trail to Barr Camp. This is Craig's weekly long run. But for me, I like to mix up the long runs with road running. Manitou Springs opens the Incline for the first time since the COVID-19 lockdowns in March and the atmosphere is different today with news reporters, volunteers, and police checking hikers' reservations. Because of the unexpected commotion, Craig and I decided to run Barr Trail, adding 1.2 miles to our route to Barr Camp. I see runners training for the Pikes Peak Marathon scheduled for August 23rd. I encounter familiar faces from the Sunrise Striders coming down the trail. They are completing today's training run and are flying downhill. The trail is covered with shredded leaves and washouts from the previous night's hailstorm. After the creek called No Name, four miles up the trail, the number of people on the trail becomes few which makes for a quiet training run. Barr Camp is another 2 miles up. When we arrive at Barr Camp, we learn that during the night it hailed golf ball-sized hail for more than half an hour. I meet the new Barr Camp caretaker, Scott, from Massachusetts. Craig orders two cups of coffee and pays two dollars per our unwritten rule that whoever reaches Barr Camp first, buys coffee. As usual, Craig arrived first. He cheated a bit, though. There's a connection between Barr Trail and the Incline, two-thirds of the way up the Incline. Craig snuck onto the Incline at this point giving him a half-mile shorter run to Barr Camp. Later this month we hike another 14er and stay overnight in Buena Vista for the ascent to the summit of Mount Yale (14,196 ft). We get up at 3:30 and begin hiking from the trailhead at 4:50. We meet two local 14er gurus, Billy and Jimmy, at the summit. It was another blissfully uneventful yet stunningly special hike up and down a 14er.

The following weekend we stay in Fairplay on Sunday night before our quad 14er hike up Mount Democrat, Mount Cameron, Mount Lincoln, and Mount Bross. We start the clockwise-direction hike at 4:45, early enough to miss the crowds. We look up into the sky and Craig points out the red planet, Mars. As soon as we start, we are lost going around the Kite Lake campground. Fifteen minutes later, after passing by several tents, we find the trailhead and begin our climb. We reach the summit of Mount Democrat and with another 2.3-mile hike, we reach the summit of Mount Cameron. I love the summit of Mount Lincoln which stands out like President Lincoln, with a sharp and distinctive summit. Mount Bross is broad with picturesque views. The hike down Mount Bross is constant mini rockslides with every step in the scree. We arrive safely back at the trailhead and drive into Fairplay for lunch and a tour of the Fairplay museum—vintage buildings along the old main street, loaded with artifacts from the mining days. Our room at the Hand Hotel gives us a river view and each room is decorated with a miner's theme, which I find fun as history intrigues me.

We summit Mount Bierstadt (14,060 ft) the next week. We drive up Guanella Pass and park in the paved parking lot (yay!)—the only paved parking lot so far other than Mount Yale. We start up the trail at 4:45. The trail seems like a highway compared to the other 14ers. At 1.5 miles, someone in front of me steps onto a side trail to adjust the load on his dog. I accidentally take the side trail, which ends up becoming a game trail leading me to a dead end with thick bushes slowing my progress for half a mile. I scream, "Craig, I am lost," but he is already too far ahead to hear me. I fall on top of a bush and start crying until I realize I can see other hikers' headlamps, which help me backtrack and find the trail. Whew. I summit Mount Bierstadt 35 minutes behind Craig. The air is smoky from several Colorado wildfires, but I can see Mount Evans in the distance. After having my snack, I start running down and feel fantastic as I pass other hikers. Suddenly, I trip and go down about a mile and a half from the parking lot. My left elbow, right knee, and right hand all have dirt mixed in with the bloody trail rash. My scraped-up body parts begin to heal when I get home and take a hot shower, but Mount Bierstadt has taught me valuable lessons:

1. When in doubt, make good decisions. If lost, return to a known location.
2. Pay attention to even the smallest rock, as that might be the one that trips you!

Our last 14er of the summer is Mount Elbert, which we climb on the final day of August. We stay overnight in

Leadville the night before and have a chance to peruse one of Leadville's many museums for another flashback to the mining days. The following day, we summit Mount Elbert, Colorado's highest mountain (14,433 ft).

I am so grateful to have had the opportunity this summer to hike from the lowest 14er, Sunshine Peak, in the San Juan Mountain Range to the highest, Mount Elbert in the Sawatch Mountain Range and so many others in between.

Summiting 14ers is as addictive as running, hooking you on the summit views and thin air. We got drawn in as soon as we climbed one. Then we had to go again... and again, and still, the next mountain is calling.

High Colorado Mountains

September 2020

<u>Crested Butte, Colorado</u>

Craig and I make an audacious overnight hiking plan. We will hike ten miles on a single-track trail from Crested Butte over West Maroon Pass to Aspen, spend the night of September 3rd in Aspen, and hike back over the pass to Crested Butte the next day. We are celebrating our sixth anniversary at the place where we were wed, Maroon Lake, Aspen. We have traveled to Europe, South America, South Africa, and Australia and Aspen is the most beautiful, magical, and romantic place we have found. We hiked and camped out on this trail a couple of years earlier and ended up hiking 13 miles each way because a snow avalanche blocked the road three miles from the Crested Butte trailhead. This year the road is clear of snow over Schofield Pass to the Crested Butte trailhead. The trailhead is at 10,432 feet, West Maroon Pass is at 12,490 feet, and the trailhead at Maroon Lake is at 9,580 feet. The weather forecast calls for perfect hiking weather with the temperature in the 40s early in the morning and warming up into the 80s. A bright full moon is right behind us as we start up the trail at 4:50. I wear my headlamp to light up the trail for both of us as Craig chose not to bring his headlamp. I packed snacks, extra socks in case of a wet stream crossing, an extra down jacket, and rain gear. After our four-hour hike to Maroon Lake, we take the bus into Aspen and check into our honeymoon suite at the Annabelle Inn, our wedding hotel. The receptionist upgraded our room since we were returning guests celebrating a special event. The inn has beautiful water features in the courtyard and colorful summer flowers surrounding the building. At 11:30 we load up with food at our favorite Aspen lunch spot, the Spring Cafe. For dinner, we indulge in a whole food plant-based meal at the Pyramid Bistro. On September 4th, we are up early and on the trail at 6:20, just as the morning is dawning. After hiking a mile, the sun is up, and the moon disappears behind Pyramid Peak. Our anniversary celebration is amazing and worth the two-day 20-mile hike. We saw a mama bear with two cubs crossing the highway on our drive to Crested Butte and bighorn sheep near West Maroon Pass. Traveling and exploring nature bestows upon us so many fresh life experiences that city life can't offer.

It has been a fun and fantastic summer without races and training, just being a free spirit enjoying the outdoors and nature in places that I would not have experienced otherwise.

Even here at home, I enjoy nature's bounty as I make my way up Barr Trail, and the warm fall sun highlights the gold and green leaves.

Exploring America the Beautiful

October 2020

<u>Poplar Bluff, Missouri</u>

October brings me triumph and sadness. Triumph with a two-week road trip and victory laps at two half marathon races. Sadness with the cancellation of the Chicago Marathon, again due to COVID-19.

Craig and I substitute the Chicago Marathon with a two-week road trip visiting eleven states together for the first time. We run two half marathon races. Our first half marathon is the Badge of Honor in Poplar Bluff, Missouri on October 10th, starting and finishing at Three River College. On the morning of the race, the sky is overcast with a chance of rain. The race officials (and we) hope it will hold off until all three scheduled races are done—5k, 10k, and half marathon. All three races start at 8:00 with cooperating weather. At mile ten, I feel a sprinkle of moisture and a soft breeze cooling my face. Because of COVID-19, the half marathon race is smaller than in past years and has 13 female finishers and 17 male finishers. As I cross the finish line, I hear the announcer say, "Here comes Hae Bolduc, the first female across the finish line in under two hours." Wow, I've never heard that before! How sweet it is to win overall female with a time of 1:58:41 and a pace of 9:06 minutes/mile.

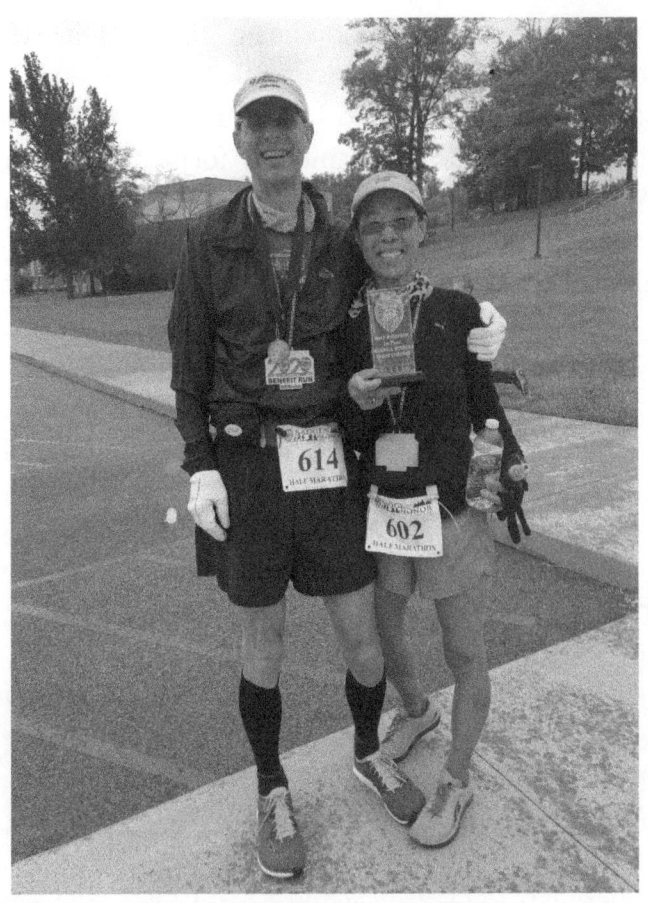

Badge of Honor First Place Female Award - Hae and Craig

Next weekend we will race in the Gettysburg, Pennsylvania Blue-Gray half marathon, which allows us time to see the sites as we drive across multiple states. We spend a night in Louisville, Kentucky in a hotel near the Ohio River waterfront. In the morning, we enjoy an easy run across the Big Four pedestrian Bridge into Jefferson, Indiana. It is a calm, pleasant morning and we take in the massiveness of the river, listening to the soft music being played on the bridge speakers.

Driving toward the northeast part of the United States is unforgettable. Virginia trees are exhibiting peak fall foliage colors and I am reminded of how much I miss the fall colors in Maine, my former home state. A visit to Thomas Jefferson's home, Monticello, is one of the highlights of our trip. Jefferson was a horticulturist with detailed notes in his gardener's logbook. Jefferson's three biggest accomplishments were writing the Declaration of Independence, founding the University of Virginia, and drafting the Virginia Statute for Religious Freedom. The next day on our drive through Shenandoah National Park, we stop and run a portion of the Appalachian Trail. We feel a sense of wonder knowing that many hikers and runners have trod on this same ground.

The day before the race we meet up with Jonathan, a former Barr Camp caretaker, and his loving Amish family. His sister, Ruthie, gave us a buggy ride and helped us experience the Amish culture of hard work, simple life, and a peaceful environment. That same morning, we meet up with other former Barr Camp caretakers, Zach, his sister Ashley, her husband Nathan, and their baby Ansel for a walk on Chickie's trail overlooking the Susquehanna River. At 444 miles long, the Susquehanna River is the longest in the Northeast and drains into the Chesapeake Bay estuary. For lunch, Craig's cousin David, from Philadelphia, meets us at the Shady Maple Smorgasbord. I feel like I'm in another world where the norm is overweight people eating a flagrant amount of overabundant buffet food. It's as if the people there don't know that overloading with oily, fatty, salty, sugary food is harmful to both their physical and mental well-being. Fortunately, we find a salad bar complete with a variety of berries to alleviate our hunger.

The Gettysburg Blue-Gray half marathon on October 18th is split into an 8:00 start group of 250 runners and a noon start group of 210 runners. We have been assigned the noon start group because of our later registration. The wind is blowing into my face and golden leaves are dancing around near the ground. The temperature is in the 60s when our wave starts. We run a portion of the race through the rolling hills of the Gettysburg National Military Park, and I can feel the long-ago anguish and torment of the fighting Blue and Gray soldiers. I finish strong with a time of 1:55:47, first in my age group out of four, shaving three minutes off my time from the previous week's race in Missouri.

We are only a four-hour drive from our granddaughter in New York but we're not able to visit them. My daughter-in-law is expecting a baby in early December and they have been cautious about minimizing contact and potential exposure to COVID-19. Since we have been around people at hotels and races, I feel obligated to keep our distance. It makes me sad not to see them, but I have been practicing Buddhism and meditation every day to detach from desires and attachments and my practice helps me cope with this separation from family. By the time we get home, Craig and I have visited for the first time together Kansas, Oklahoma, Missouri, Kentucky, Indiana, West Virginia, Virginia, Pennsylvania, Illinois, Ohio, and Maryland. I experienced much beauty in this land I call home, America!

New Birth

November 2020

<u>Colorado Springs</u>

Our second granddaughter, Zaydee Christopher (after her grandfather's name) Cartagena Bolduc, arrives early and is born on November 1st.

Yin and Yang is the Chinese notion of dualism, the idea that seemingly opposite or contrary forces may be complementary, interconnected, and interdependent in the natural world. Consider the cycle of life and death. While that little life is entering the world, we also experience the death of a friend's family member. Steve Jobs said, "No one wants to die. Even people who want to go to heaven don't want to die to get there. And yet death is the destination we all share. No one has ever escaped it. And that is as it should be because death is very likely the single best invention of life. It is life's change agent. It clears out the old to make way for the new."

The morning is a dark and calm 19°F at 6:10 when I put on my headlamp and head out the door to do hill repeats on Steep Mother. I witness an amazing contrast as the moon is about to disappear behind the foothills to the west and the welcoming sun begins to rise from the east. When I run, I experience and appreciate the Yin and Yang in the beauty of opposing scenery.

Solemnity

December 2020

<u>Cajun Country, Louisiana</u>

We fly to Lafayette, Louisiana for our last race of the year, the Cajun Country half marathon on December 12th.

I run a 1:54:58 and take home the grandmaster (over 50 years old) winner's trophy complete with a baby alligator head (yes, a real one) nailed onto it. We spend the better part of a day in New Orleans visiting the sites before returning home.

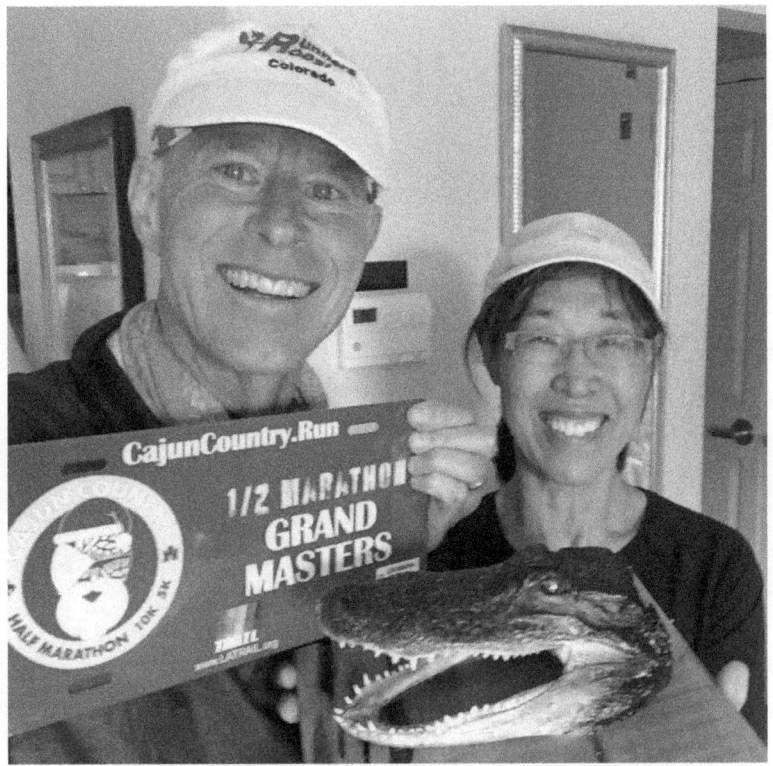

Hae's First Place Grand Master Trophy

There is still no COVID-19 end in sight. Nonetheless, we have had an amazing year traveling 20 new states together, climbing fourteen 14ers, and running five races in different states despite restrictions and missed visits with family and friends. Now Zoom rather than in-person meetings seems normal. Everyone has their eye on a vaccine to end this pandemic and hopefully put an end to mask-wearing. It's odd not seeing people's expressions with mask-covered faces. I miss the simple human touch of hugging when I run into my friends at the market. Life feels strange in these never-before-experienced times.

2021

New Year, New Goals
Spring—March 2021
<u>Colorado Springs</u>

Spring arrives with six inches of wet, sloppy snow. My coach has put together my training schedule for 2021 which includes three marathons. The first is REVEL Sun Valley, Idaho on June 26th. This is a downhill race starting at 7,834 feet and finishing at 5,799 feet for a net elevation drop of 2,035 feet. My goals for this race are as follows:

1. Finish with a time under four hours.
2. Set a new personal record (PR).
3. Place first in my age group.

The other two big ones are part of the six major world marathons, the Chicago Marathon, October 10th, and the New York City Marathon, November 7th. Since I missed out on both last year due to COVID-19 cancellations, I'm very hopeful that I'll be able to run both of them this year. If so, my goals for these two marathons are to run well, finish, and have fun.

I am running my favorite workout today, hill repeats, on Steep Mother. The snow slows me down to over two minutes up the hill (2:14). During my training for Boston, without the snow, my best time up this hill was 1:30.

Resilience

Summer—June 2021

Colorado Springs and Sun Valley, ID

The sweetest email ever just arrived from the New York City Marathon with the opening words "Congratulations, you're in." It has been more than two long years since I was first accepted and I have been training hard for the 50th anniversary of this prestigious race. I am determined to run it on November 7th.

The sweet, strong fragrance of Russian Olive trees along the trail is heavenly this morning. The temperature is already in the 60s at 5:30. I am running an easy, short run before our upcoming Sun Valley Marathon. I am thrilled to see in-person races taking place again and a return to near normalcy in the racing world. After weeks of blistering heat, nature cooled us with rain last night. The tall, green grass is quenching its thirst, smiling, and tickling my legs as I run past on the single-track trail. Inhaling fresh, cool air awakens my body as I run up and down the hills in a familiar course around the neighborhood. I am so grateful to be running and enjoying the fresh air. I try to never take for granted small things, even something as simple as the air I breathe.

We lay out our running clothes, socks, and bibs, and have breakfast ready to go the night before the Sun Valley Marathon. We wake up at 3:05 on race day. I eat my pre-race breakfast of coffee, toast with peanut butter, and a banana. I dress in my race shorts and shirt and put on my Altra Escalante race shoes. Because the forecast predicts a hot day, the race director moved the starting times ahead by 40 minutes. Our start time is now 6:10. We park our car in the dark parking lot and load the race bus. After getting off the bus, we have five minutes to line up for the start of our wave. Only a five-minute wait—that's a first! We are surrounded by mountains shading the sun at a very comfortable 50°F, with no wind.

Starting at Galena Pass on Highway 75, the initial three miles have the steepest downhill grade and offer a fun way to start the race. At mile 14, the sun comes out from behind the mountains as the downhill grade lessens. Aid stations are spaced approximately three miles apart, and I drink water at each one. I fuel with the same easily digestible Maurten gels I have been training with. While focusing on each step and each mile, I see the time of 3:05 on the clock at mile 20. I quickly calculate that I might be able to break four hours if I just "kick it into high gear." Deep down, though, I know that my first goal of breaking four hours is beginning to slip by. At mile 22, I catch up with Craig, who is barely moving. I say, "Hi," and he yells back, "Keep going." I finish with a time of 4:11:35. At 4:30 on the clock, Craig crosses the finish line. He is exhausted. I meet him and help hold him up. The outside temperature is nearly 80°F, and we later determined he became overheated during the second half of the race. When we get back home, we start "heat training" with 30-minute sessions in the sauna in preparation for the Chicago Marathon.

Healthy, Fit, and Rested

Fall—October 2021

<u>Chicago, Illinois</u>

On October 10th, 2021, at the start of the Chicago Marathon, I line up with 35,000 other runners. I feel like I'm in the Olympics. In what other sport can you line up with the elites, pros, and highest-level amateurs? Yes, I am half a mile behind the starting line and the elite runners, but we are all running the SAME 26.2 miles.

The Chicago Marathon has a dangerous element to it this year, with both high temperature and humidity. The race starts with a yellow warning and a temperature of 74°F. My qualifying time is slower than Craig's so I have a start time of 8:10 a.m. in corral H. Craig's start time is 7:30 in corral E. Since Craig is in the back of the first wave and I am in the middle of the second wave, we cross the starting line only 20 minutes apart. We wish each other good luck before going to our separate corrals. Note to self—next time I should bring my phone. It's a bit heavy but good to have for emergencies like injury or heat exhaustion where my mind could play tricks on me.

I am ready. I have put in my training and show up at the starting line fit, healthy, and rested. My thought of chasing a sub-four-hour finish time means nothing to anyone except me. But then again, we should always be struggling to know who we are and what we are capable of.

By noon the temperature was in the 80s, a red flag warning and a chance the officials could stop the race. EMTs are all over the sidelines, helping the runners who are dropping out like flies. When my "wheels come off" around mile 15, I drop my hopes for finishing in under four hours and concentrate on my goals for the race—run well, finish, and have fun. Success is not about a particular finish time when the weather or other factors make it risky. For myself, the 1.5 million spectators, and the twenty thousand volunteers who give us so much while running through the streets of Chicago, I dig deep and finish with a time of 4:28:44. Craig had a rough time in the heat. After finishing, I waited in the hotel for an hour and a half before Craig showed up. After the effort and turmoil of completing the Chicago Marathon, I slept with the finisher's medal for several days. The Chicago Marathon was hot and grueling, yet it was one of the most beautiful days of my life.

Finally!
Fall—November 2021
New York City, New York

The big day is approaching fast. A couple of weeks before race day, I receive an email with my bib number, wave and corral, bus loading location, and race day schedule. During my week's rest after the Chicago Marathon, I realize just how much I have learned. The New York City Marathon will be my fun marathon, for once. I don't plan to look at my watch or be concerned with my pace.

I am looking forward to my best marathon ever. My kids and grandkids live an hour away, and I will be running through five boroughs in a magical city with beautiful people, high-energy ambiance, and Broadway shows. My goal is to have fun while running.

I have four weeks between the Chicago Marathon and the New York City Marathon. My first slow recovery jog is four days after the Chicago Marathon. I monitor my body and practice not looking at my watch. I have been stretching a lot and working on my legs with a foam roller. My legs feel great during the run, and I'm amazed at how resilient my body is. I've recovered quickly and feel like Chicago never happened.

Friday morning before the New York City Marathon, the alarm startles me out of a deep sleep at 3:45. My small backpack is packed and my food bag is waiting for me in the fridge. We are flying from Colorado Springs to La Guardia with a layover in Denver. I have been waiting to run this marathon since 2019. In 2019 I felt like I was at peak fitness after running the Boston Marathon in April and training at a higher intensity leading up to the New York City Marathon. This year, the quality and quantity of training are equal to 2019, but could two years later be a factor?

On the airplane from Denver to La Guardia, a beautiful sunrise appears on the horizon. I am filled with excitement and energy. After leaving the terminal at La Guardia airport, we catch the Q70 bus to Jackson Heights/Roosevelt Ave. and transfer to the subway for our ride to downtown Manhattan and our hotel for three nights. Craig has again been a detailed and excellent travel agent. We are staying at a Hilton hotel close to the pre-race bus pickup location and close to the marathon finish line.

Race Preparation

Saturday, November 6th

<u>New York City, New York</u>

Early Saturday morning Craig and I run 0.5 miles from our hotel to Central Park and one mile in the park as part of my 2-mile shakeout run. I see race officials working on the barricades and the finish line with timing mats and spectator stands. Many other runners are also out doing their final pre-marathon run anticipating the big day. Craig and I decide to meet after the marathon at the iconic Columbia Circle, at the southwest corner of Central Park.

We walk 1.2 miles from our hotel to the Javits Center to pick up my bib at 10:00. You must be vaccinated or provide proof of a negative COVID-19 test to go into the Javits Center building, otherwise, you are allowed to pick up your bib at an outside location and miss the indoor expo. The marathon event planner did an outstanding job coordinating the bib pickup, and I received mine without waiting.

In the evening, I eat my Leafside lentil pasta meal brought from home. Craig reserved a room with a microwave oven, so I just add water to the lentil pasta in our Pyrex bowl and cook it for five minutes. I have eaten this pre-race lentil pasta at both the Sun Valley and Chicago marathons without issues, so I stick with a proven pre-race dinner. I lay out my running shorts and shirt with my bib attached. Tomorrow morning I'll eat my usual long-run breakfast, also brought from home, coffee and toast with peanut butter and banana. My Spring Energy gels are packed into my running belt in the order I plan to eat them—mile 10 - CanaBerry, mile 15 - Long Haul, mile 20 - Speed Nut, and mile 24 - CanaBerry. I also made a half sandwich with peanut butter and banana to fuel my six-hour wait from the time I leave the hotel until I start racing. We watch a light comedy movie in the evening to minimize the jittery anticipation of tomorrow's run.

Race Day

Sunday, November 7th

New York City, New York

I get up at 4:30 before either of our phone alarms goes off. I eat my toast and drink my coffee. We leave the hotel room at 5:25 and walk the half mile to Bryant Park where I will catch the bus to Staten Island.

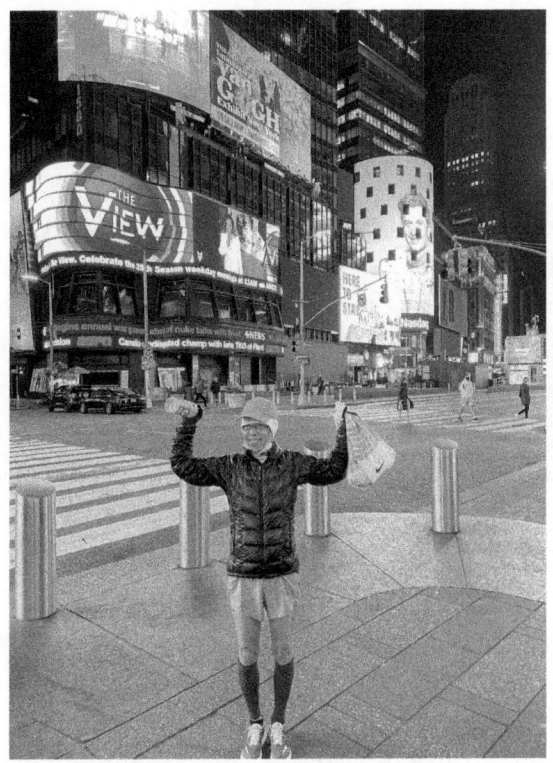

Hae on the Walk to Bryant Park

When we get to Bryant Park, runners are lined up and wrapped in blankets, pajamas, hats, and gloves. The line to the buses moves quickly. Craig accompanies me in the line for as long as possible. We kiss and say goodbye. I won't see him again until mile 15 after crossing the Queensboro Bridge into Manhattan, more than seven hours later.

The New York City Marathon is epic and unlike any other marathon. The Star-Spangled Banner is played for the start of each wave of runners, and I hear it as I begin my own 26.2-mile journey. The view of the city from the Verrazano Bridge is incredible and I get choked up when I hear Frank Sinatra's "New York, New York" as I run across the bridge from Staten Island to Brooklyn. With the Brooklyn spectators cheering, music playing in Queens and the Bronx, and the loud crowd lining Central Park, I run without effort.

I had taped my name onto the front and back of my shirt and was cheered on, by name and with high fives, by hundreds of the 2.5 million spectators. It's an amazing experience to feel the energy of the city and hear the cheering. When I see a spectator with a sign reading, "Run a mile for someone who could not run," I get emotional, and tears flow down my cheeks. The sign inspires an energy boost and I do my best to run that mile for someone who can't.

I see Craig at mile 15 after coming down into Manhattan from the Queensboro Bridge. I give him a quick kiss and continue. The crowds at this point are going crazy and encroaching on the racecourse. I give the closest spectators high fives. They are chanting, "Let's go Hae." I am smiling and crying at the same time. I am in the moment with the other runners, taking it all in. I am so grateful for all the runners, the crowds, the supportive families, my husband and coach, friends, race officials, the New York City Police, and all the volunteers. This is an amazing and unbelievable experience.

I can see the finish line and hear the crowd roar. I cross the finish line with a time of 4:28:42. With my tired legs, my mind is empty of thoughts. I try to spot Craig among the seemingly endless runners and families where we are supposed to meet at Columbia Circle. I don't see Craig at Columbia Circle, and slowly begin wandering to the hotel. Suddenly, out of nowhere Craig shows up and gives me a big hug and kiss with a huge smile on his face. He congratulates me. What a feeling of accomplishment and victory! I achieved my goals for the marathon—run well, finish, and have fun—by more than I ever dreamed.

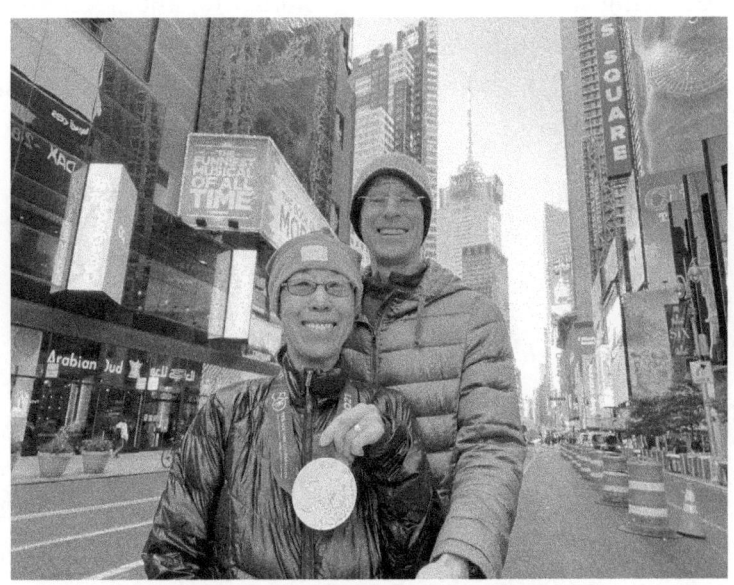

Hae Beaming with Her New York City
Marathon Finisher's Medal

To top off the experience, on the short return-home flight from Denver to Colorado Springs, I sit next to Elkanah Kibet, the fastest United States runner in the New York City Marathon finishing fourth overall. He is on the US

Army running team and stationed in Colorado Springs. He gave me some great marathon training tips. Stretch after every run. Run 22, 20, and 22 miles for the three long runs building up to a marathon. And going into the fourth week before the race, taper with 18, 16, and 14-mile long runs on flat routes. Awesome advice I plan to follow.

Back home, at last, I celebrate with a cup of coffee and feel immense gratitude to the Pikes Peak Road Runners, who I trained with and who motivated me to run my best. I get congratulations from all my neighbors and friends when I see them during my post-marathon jogs. Life is all about celebrating little successes, big moments, and seemingly impossible accomplishments and these past three years have had some of each. I feel serene and in awe, as I close my final chapter of running the New York City Marathon.

2022

Epilogue

2022 has been a fantastic running year for me. I have run 14 races—already more than any previous year—as I finish up the book for a July publication. I will start ramping up my training for the Berlin marathon in the fall. But let me go back to these races and give you an update on my performance.

Rescue Run - Jan 1, 10k, 1st place age group (1:04:40), Snow covered hilly trails, 6°F.

Winter Series I - Jan 8, 10k, 1st place age group (1:00:09)

Winter Series II - Jan 22, 8m, 1st place age group (1:28:24), very hilly single track trail

Big Ocean (Gulf Shores, AL) - Jan 30, half marathon, 1st place age group (2:00:16)

Winter Series III - Feb 5, 10m, 1st place age group (1:38:34)

Super Half Marathon - Feb 13, half marathon, 3rd place age group (2:04:35)

Winter Series IV - Feb 19, 12m, 1st place age group (1:44:46)

Pueblo Spring Runoff (Pueblo, CO) - Mar 5, 10m, 1st place age group (1:34:02)

St. Patrick's Day 5k - Mar 12, 5k, 2nd place age group (27:36)

Mt. Charleston Marathon (Las Vegas, NV) - Apr 2, marathon, 1st place age group (3:45:06) Mt. Charleston is located in Clark County, Nevada and the peak is at 11,916 feet. The full marathon starts at 7,633 feet and finishes at 2,507 feet for a net elevation drop of 5,126 feet. This was an epic race for me—MY FIRST MARATHON UNDER 4 HOURS AND A PERSONAL RECORD BY 15 MINUTES!!

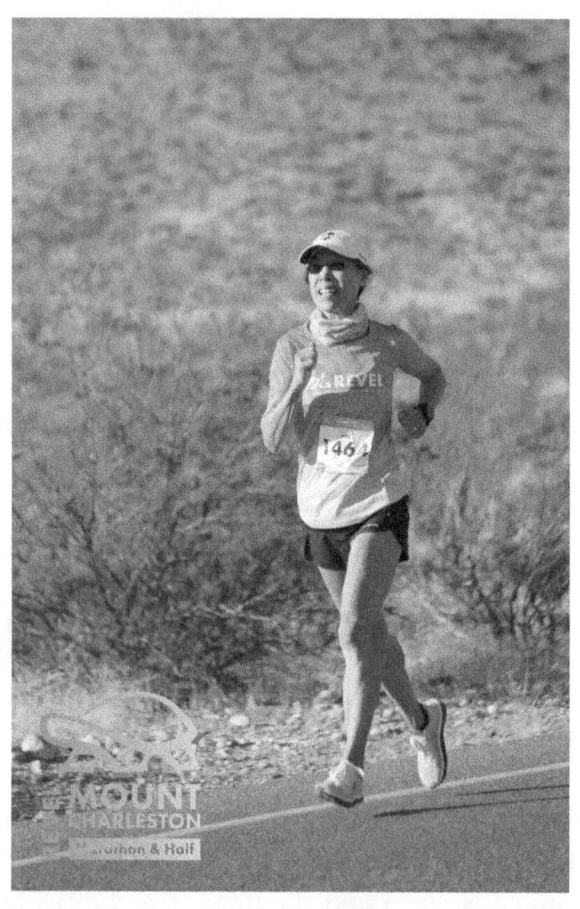

Mount Charleston Running to a New Personal Record

La Crosse, WI Marathon - May 7, 1st place age group (4:05:48) ANOTHER HUGE ACCOMPLISHMENT—FASTEST FLAT MARATHON! I created an account with Abbott World Marathon Majors and for $15 I could compete on May 7th or 8th for one of 100 women's masters division entries to the Abbott World Marathon Majors Wanda Age Group Championships. I placed 29th and earned an entry. I have now been invited to compete in the London Marathon, October 2nd, 2022. I am so excited for the opportunity, but on the other hand I am running the Berlin Marathon on September 25th. After much deliberation, the coach suggested I run both. I know that time does not wait for us, so I am going for it.

Bolder Boulder - May 30, 10k, 4th place age group (56:40)

Garden of the Gods - Jun 11, 10m, 1st place age group (1:38:07)

Mt Evans - Jun 26, 14.5m, 1st place age group (3:38:16), The race starts at 10,600 feet and with a vertical gain of 3,600 feet, finishes at the summit of Mt Evans at 14,264 feet.

I have been having so much fun this year, training and racing. It has been an amazing year running so many races. The Berlin Marathon and the London Marathon are two of the "biggies," two of the six major world marathons. I am excited to train for and run these marathons. Once again, running provides me simplicity, pureness, and honesty. Whatever I put into running, I get back, many times over. Running completes me with social activity, new friendships, health, fitness, endorphins, and fun results! I am so grateful for my ability to run, for my family, friends, my husband, my health, a beautiful life—for everything.

Lightning Source UK Ltd.
Milton Keynes UK
UKHW041825041122
411674UK00008B/163/J